CLEANSE INTERNALLY

Controversies, Benefits, and Facts

By

Millan Chessman

Printed in the United States of America.

Library of Congress Control Number: 2011961893

ISBN # 978-0-9834722-0-9

Published by

NUTRITION FACTS PUBLISHER
2633 Windmill View Rd.
El Cajon, Ca. 92020
millanchessman@gmail.com

TABLE OF CONTENTS

ACKNOWLEDGEMENTS

I want to thank William Saccoman, M.D., of El Cajon, California, who had confidence in me and allowed me to work out of his office, giving me my start in internal cleansing.

Thank you, Leslie Williams, former President of the International Association for Colon hydrotherapy (I-ACT), for contributing your wisdom and research.

Sam Warren (Bookwarren Publishing Services), I could not have done this book without your help. You were always there for me. I am humbly grateful for all your expertise.

INTRODUCTION

What if you found out that a few minor adjustments to your diet and lifestyle, coupled with a simple, painless, and inexpensive office procedure, could help you not only live longer, but maintain ultimate health, vigor and mental acuity into your nineties and beyond?

Would you take the necessary steps to enjoy life unimpaired, especially if these steps were low-cost, low-tech, drug-free, and non-strenuous? Does this sound too good to be true? NO!

Chances are your doctor will not tell you how to take these steps. He or she probably does not know about them.

These pages reveal the answer to optimum health.

Wouldn't it be great not to rely on expensive doctors, high-tech equipment, drugs, and hospitals?

A healthy person does not need to rely on medical help. The answer to ultimate youthfulness and health is internal cleansing. So many have benefited from this simple and painless procedure.

If we want to be healthier, live longer, and improve our outlook, we need to examine the vital core of our well-being. This core is finally becoming obvious to more than an elite few who have known for years that a key to health is in the colon.

I believe that internal cleansing is vital to optimum health. In the past 30 years, more health practitioners than ever before have advocated internal cleansing.

5

When you consider that the average American consumes 1 pound of food additives per year, and there are over 3,000 toxic chemicals we are ingesting, one realizes the absolute necessity of internal cleansing.

In the following pages, actual personal testimonies will describe the relief others received from pain and illness through internal cleansing programs. These testimonials were collected over the years from my own practice. I hope they, along with the information in this book, will inspire you to take charge of your life by taking charge of your health through internal cleansing.

A complete cleansing program includes either fasting or diet modification. This provides the start to continue a client's newfound health.

This therapy is seldom mentioned in modern medical literature, and what happens to be cited is overwhelmingly negative. Without factual basis, the literature presents internal cleansing as useless and unfounded. Its overarching importance to health is grossly overlooked and ignored.

Testimonial

Old unhealthy Habits Gone

Dear Millan:

I wasn't experiencing any major problems when I started the sessions. This wasn't to say that I felt like a million bucks, or that my diet was pure as the driven snow. After the first cleansing, I immediately felt different. As the sessions went on, I was amazed at the changes taking place in my body. After a few cleansings, there was no way I could go back to my old habits. I truly did not realize the shape I was in. Since then, I have felt a feeling of overwhelming good health.

I have cleaned my lifestyle considerably. Thank you for your information and expertise.

Jason O.

CHAPTER ONE

Quote: We can touch the lives of our fellow man, on our path of life and can influence greatly for better or worse. That is our power and they can be forever changed. Millan Chessman

HISTORY OF INTERNAL CLEANSING

Internal cleansing is an ancient health treatment. Historically, it has been used successfully to treat almost every condition imaginable. But today, orthodox medical opinion takes a dim view of internal cleansing. Even enemas are suspect, though for certain medical conditions and procedural preparations - colonoscopy, lower GI X-rays, prep for many surgeries, and childbirth – enemas are still employed.

Origin of Colon Cleansing
Four-thousand-year-old Egyptian artifacts depict enema implements and their uses. One document, known as the Ebers Papyrus, a toxicological and medical text by priests circa 1552 B.C., describes the procedure of "colon lavage."

Egyptians credited colon cleansing's origin to a legendary bird, the sacred ibis. Stork-like, with a downward-curved bill, the sacred ibis was said to have invented colon cleansing when, it seemed, it injected water from its bill into its own bowel. Colon cleansing thus involved rectally infusing certain "aqueous substances" - there were then an array of usable solutions - into the large intestine.

Past Cultures

There is some indication in past cultures this particular bodily function and its product were not considered offensive, or at least not compared to today. The putrid odor makes it currently offensive.

In ancient Japan, public contests were held to see who could break wind loudest and longest. Winners were awarded many prizes and received great acclaim.

We have come a long way since then!

I am sure their gas was not offensive, because otherwise they certainly would not be public heroes; people would run the opposite direction. This shows in earlier days there was nothing disgusting or shameful about their lower digestive system.

Dark Ages

Historically, colon cleansing has been used to purge the large intestine.

During the Dark Ages, the technique's greatest employments were to counteract poisons (which were the most popular ways to commit murder or assassination) and to fight disease. Identification of poisons, plaques, and food poisoning (from rotting meats and other foods) was almost impossible to determine, so colon cleansing was used extensively.

Though many kinds of colon cleansings were described and used for centuries, it was not until 1600 A.D. that Dr. Pare distinguished the difference between colon hydrotherapy and "the popular enema of the day."

After this, the course of colon cleansings proves harder to track. Perhaps because in our culture the subject is publicly taboo, records of internal cleansing in the last two hundred years are rare. Some records may be found under the headings of physical therapy or massage. These were the areas of application until turf wars with the

8

medical profession removed those avenues of application.

In 500 B.C., Hippocrates, the Greek father of modern medicine, used colon cleansing to bring fevers down. This remains a valid application. Another Greek physician, Galen, also administered colon cleansing to his patients and wrote about its uses in 200 A.D. These doctors both used colon cleansing in their practices.

Royal Cleansings

In Europe, colon cleansing was common, especially among royalty. In eighteenth century France, "enema stools" were as common as footstools. "Colon laundries" were even established in London.

Before refrigeration, food spoiled quickly. Rich, flavorful sauces and gravies enjoyed today were created in ancient times to mask the taste and odor of putrefying food. For the wealthy, who could afford meat on a regular basis, it was not unusual to follow dinner with a colon cleansing.

J. Glenn Knox, D.C., states:

For thousands of years most health practitioners were actually midwives and "lay nurses." These medicine women, healers, the wise women of their tribes and villages, used colon cleansing and combined it with herbs and massages.

From observing their patients, these women knew the health benefits of a clean, unclogged digestive system. They rightly believed a toxic body caused many illnesses.

Dierken - One of the Original Colonic Equipments

Dierken Therapeutic Apparatus is one of the oldest known types of colon cleansing equipment.

Figure one

Figure one shows antique colonic equipment.

Figure two shows professional colon hydrotherapy system, new safety and sanitation features that greatly improved efficacy of the treatment.

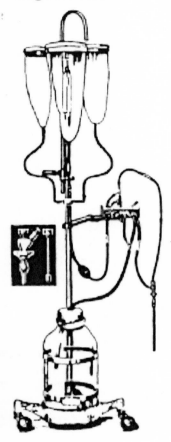

In 1940, this machine was a considerable improvement over other types. It had, its promoters pointed out, "the effect of promoting physiological peristalsis, and of working free the contents of the 'pockets' and diverticula."

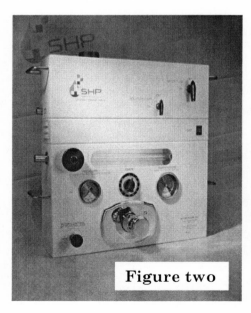

Figure two

The Dierken machine had "a glass percolator and all the necessary plumbing attachments, control valves, and special irrigation features compactly assembled within a stainless steel alloy frame."

Present History

Internal cleansing has been used for centuries; however, only in present history has it become one of the most silenced topics of discussion among the lay public and its doctors. It is ironic this is the case now, when internal cleansing is needed in the most toxic time in our history.

Technological Advances

Increased technological requirements in education changed the titles of the "players." The "hospitals," where patients were treated, became the proper "stage" for treatment. By the late 1800's, modern science rapidly grew in organized fields of study. These were initiated and taken over by men for religious reasons, prestige, dominance, control, and monetary gain. These men became the doctors, and the common midwife became the nurse.

While it was not unseemly for mothers or nurses to administer enemas, more and more doctors disdained performing the procedure. After all, why spend years learning the marvels of the human body only to end up dealing with feces and offensive odors from patients unable to hold water in their colons?

So, the enema bags and internal cleansing equipment used in most hospitals until the 1950's (though not standard procedure as in earlier times) were relegated to nurses. And later, doctors passed bowel treatment administration onto others.

Keeping the patient's colon cleansed was the main duty of the attending nurses. Colon cleansing was ever-present, and patients received treatment during most hospital stays.

Testimonial

Into the 20th Century

As doctors gained power through medical breakthroughs, their services came at higher prices.

With the birth of the Industrial Age in the late 1800's, the art of medicine became a thriving enterprise, reflecting the success rate of many large-scale businesses and factories.

In the first decades of the 20th century, standardized accreditation requirements were instituted for medical schools. This reduced the number of approved medical teaching schools.

Consequently, the social and financial position of physicians increased.

No More Messy Procedures

Through the years, internal cleansing has undergone many changes. Conventional medicine began to drop archaic, messy procedures, such as colon cleansing as practiced prior to the 1950's.

The Western world entered the age of surgery, medications, and pills with rejoicing and awe. Fantastic - no need for repugnant, time-consuming colon cleansing.

Just prescribe a pill - and keep your hands clean - to get rid of unwelcome diseases.

Flourishing a pen, a doctor would prescribe quick, painless prescription drugs, usually solving the patient's problem - at least for the short term.

Meanwhile, the value of clean bowels was slowly dismissed. After all, who wanted to spend time, with little financial reward, dealing with the lower digestive system of the body.

Safe Equipment

Today we have state-of-the-art, safe equipment with sanitation features, disposable speculums and tubing, and highly trained, certified colon hydrotherapists. The medical community that once banned internal cleansing should now recognize and incorporate modern internal cleansing into any complete health program.

Testimonial

Life Changing Experience

Dear Millan:

I have been in ministry for the last 15 years and I can count on one-hand ministries that delivered life-defining experiences for me. Yours is definitely one of them. Your merciful and gracious spirit, your healing hands and excellent program has literally transformed the way I live.

I have been experiencing new levels of energy, acuity and focus.

My meditation and prayer times are deeper and I am excited about the benefits Aileen and I are sharing as a couple. We look forward to staying connected to you the rest of our lives.

Many Thanks,
Daniel T.

CHAPTER TWO

Quote: Planning is bringing the future to present to proceed with action. Millan Chessman

MY STORY

My first internal cleansing was in 1972. When I saw what came out of my young, beautiful, and perfect body or so I thought, I was shocked. I thought, "If I contain such garbage, then other people must also!"

I read every health, nutrition, and internal cleansing book I could get my hands on. My elimination took place once every five or six days. I knew this was not ideal, but my medical doctor said it was "normal" for me.

You may have heard that yourself.

My personal and professional research and experience have taught me emphatically it is not normal for me, or anybody else, to walk around carrying rotting pounds of sewage in the body for weeks and even years.

Some health practitioners believe that because the average American could have five to fifteen and more pounds of fecal matter in the colon, havoc is played with the body's balance of intake and elimination. This is the reason behind many potbellies. Granted, fat is there, but excess stool is definitely there as well.

This, in reality, makes us walking cesspools and an open invitation to disease and sickness.

I am greatly concerned and want the public to know there is hope beyond health problems.

Many years ago, I had a class-two Pap smear and the nurses and doctor frightened me into getting this problem treated immediately, or I would end up with cancer of the uterus.

I then went to three different gynecologists, and they all said I needed a hysterectomy. Some authorities believe eighty-five percent of all such surgeries are unnecessary. I refused to let them cut into my body, and ultimately had the area in question cauterized by another doctor. It was the most painful procedure, and my knees began to knock together as my body went into shock. After the doctor was finished, I uncontrollably began to cry. I could not explain why I was crying so violently.

About seven years later, I had another class-two Pap smear; again, the threat of ultimate cancer. This time I went on a seven-day fast, drinking only organic, fresh juices, taking cleansing herbs, and did colonics each day for the week.

In the meantime, the doctor's office kept phoning me with great urgency to come in for treatment. I completed the fast, went back to the doctor, and had another pap test done.

THIS ONE CAME OUT NEGATIVE!

My doctor and nurses were shocked and, in light of the previous positive Pap smears, could not understand what had happened. I told them what I had done, and they said absolutely nothing to me. They did not even want to discuss this any further.

I provide this personal example to be an encouragement to you.

I attended the Arizona Wholistic Institute, where I learned anatomy, physiology, nutrition, and health. While there, I also learned how the digestive system interacts with all other body systems, the important psychological implications, and how to administer internal cleansing.

16

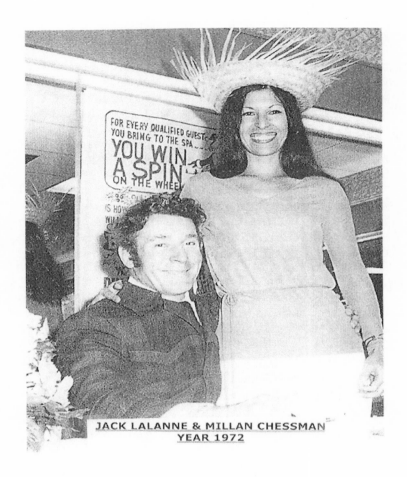

JACK LALANNE & MILLAN CHESSMAN
YEAR 1972

Terms for this procedure are entero lavage, colonic, colon therapy, or internal cleansing. All of these terms mean cleansing the body, primarily the colon. I am correctly referred to as a colon hydrotherapist.

I am now considered a pioneer with thirty years experience in the fasting/detox industry, as of the writing of this book.

I read every book possible about fasting, cleansing, and enemas. However, most of my experience comes from my years of practice.

Putting Forth the Effort

Cleansing our bodies and eating the foods God intended for us to eat is the very simple answer. Rome was not built in a day. Not all the years of abuse done to one's body will be remedied with a quick fix or a pill. We have to be patient, determined, and persevere.

What is great is that the results are for everyone! Unfortunately, many people clean out their bodies and go back to old eating habits.

One client told me, "If I can't have my beer and steak, I'd rather be dead."

I saw this man only once and he is no longer around. Another man had prostate cancer but was unwilling to give up his cigarettes and steaks. He died just recently.

You see, there is no easy way.

There is a perfect plan for good health and longevity. Balance is required in this plan; of equal weight are a godly diet, exercise, and a clean body.

You may have heard it said that you do not appreciate something until you do not have it. That really applies to health, vitality, and youth. We take these things for granted.

As a young teenager seeing old people, I remember thinking, "I will never look like that. Not me!"

Can you imagine the foolishness of my mind? I honestly thought I would be young forever.

Let me tell you, I never exercised a day in my life until I turned fifty. I was determined to keep a youthful figure. I always thought exercise was for those unfortunates with weight problems or something.

I hated the thought of exercise!

But look at me now! I am like the horse in the starting gate. I cannot wait to get to my aerobics class. I am here to tell you that once one has been unhealthy and sick, and then cleansed the body, how one feels and looks afterwards is more valuable than gold. At age 72, I am now a licensed Zumba instructor.

More than that, all the effort and perseverance is worth its weight in gold, ten times over. One is never the same, not ever wanting to go back to old ways. It just is not worth it.

I cannot and do not serve a God who expects me to grow old, sick, and in pain! Granted, I will be growing old; however, how I grow old is very important to me.

I want to grow old healthy. I want to be an asset not a burden to my immediate family.

Take control of your health. Physical perfection is for you. Do not settle for anything less. Examine all the facts and search out the truth. An informed decision is the only way.

Likewise, our bodies are capable of functioning in a manner far superior to what we are experiencing.

We each are given only one body, so let us take control of it, and give it what it needs, not what it wants. I am not saying we will always be squeaky clean. That is very improbable in our culture, where food is often the center of social gatherings.

When we do blow it, don't continue eating the wrong foods. When that happens, my clients take about twelve wheat grass tablets with two glasses of distilled water or super aloe capsules with two glasses of distilled water.

This procedure flushes most bad food, so clients feel much better and soon get back on the right track again.

Testimonial

Waste Removed Cleared Health Problems

Dear Millan:

Never in my wildest dreams did I ever imagine that my body could harbor such tremendous amounts of garbage.

I developed terrible pains in my stomach and all across my abdomen. It kept me awake all night.

I decided to see an alternative Medical Doctor. She suggested I visit you and do your seven day supervised fasting and colonics program.

I watched my colon being cleansed of tremendous amounts of fecal matter-sewage-garbage. With yours and God's help wonderful results occurred. I am now able to sleep without any pain. For years I had arthritis in both thumbs of my hand. It hurt terribly when I would hold a pencil, or try to grip anything. Now that is completely gone. I can now hold and grip without the excruciating pain. Before I came to you, I would get up in the morning and my eyes would be almost sticky and difficult to open. That has cleared up completely. I am thankful and grateful to you and bless the day I met you and the wonderful internal cleansings that I have done. Your cleansing program is far superior to any that is available. God bless and thank you.

Signed,
Robert P.

Life-changing Program

I have worked in San Diego as a certified colon hydrotherapist since 1982. My experience, after administering over twenty five thousand internal cleansing sessions, and relieving much pain and anguish, has compelled me to publicize the need for individuals to start internal cleansing. Internal cleansing will truly change lives.

When my clients see all kinds of rotten matter come out of their bodies, they experience what I call a "new awakening," and their lives are never the same.

When I first established my internal cleansing practice, I was under the supervision of William Saccoman, M.D. My approach has been different from many other colon hydrotherapists.

20

Whereas internal cleansing is the beginning and end of most practices, my services include *the Cadillac of all cleansing programs*: a complete program of providing information on the many benefits of green smoothies and eating correctly.

CHAPTER THREE

Quote: Realize your health is wealth and will affect you and your loved ones.
Millan Chessman

CULTURAL AND SOCIAL ATTITUDES

Many Medical doctors tend to avoid anything pertaining to the colon. Perhaps some find the subject offensive and below their dignity and training.

In the morning, if your boss comes into the office grumpy, could it be because his bowels did not move?

Discussion relating to bowel movements should not be considered "offensive," yet this is the case in our culture. By contrast, all areas of sex are discussed openly, with no embarrassment. Sex was also an "unspeakable" only thirty years ago, considered unfit for polite conversation. It was a private, very personal and intimate subject.

The recent sexual revolution is due largely to educational efforts, such as sex-education in classrooms, and wide exposure through the media.

Open discussion of bowel habits, conditions, and contents is still a taboo subject in our culture.

Once, in a TV interview, when I started discussing bowel movement, the host of the program actually started squirming and making the funniest faces. But wouldn't you know, the station's phone rang off the hook after that show, all from people wanting more information about internal cleansing.

During the Roman Empire, Romans not only had bathhouses but also social toilets. These so-

23

cial toilets were lounge benches with holes in them. Folks sat and visited while they defecated. This may indicate that their bowel movements did not have an offensive odor; certainly, their normal diet was high in fiber-plant foods.

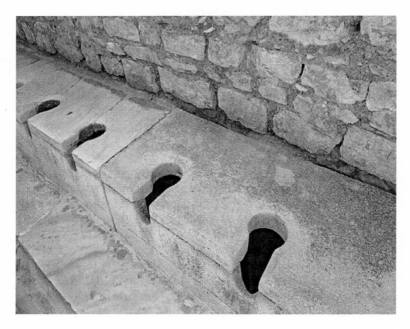

This photo of a "social toilet" was taken in ancient Ephesus.

In today's day the lower part of the digestive system is a difficult subject to discuss. We can speak with ease about what goes into the mouth and into the stomach, but conversation stops there. Food is digested through the stomach and small intestine, but what happens from that point on is usually ignored or avoided.

A Simple Solution
Bowel movements of breast-fed infants have no offensive odor. Adult stools should be that way, and can be, if we clean out our presently polluted colon and eat God-made foods.

24

People accept without question - yet equally without substantiation – that everything medically possible is being done to find cures and other alleviating treatments for the diseases plaguing us daily. Supposedly, our best interest is the concern. All avenues are explored and clues followed on the cause and ultimate destruction of disease, so that all humankind – or at least, all Americans – can finally live disease free. But this is not happening.

Colon research and its direct relationship to disease and health are not being researched by the great institutions in our country.

The ultimate solution is simple and cheap, internal cleansing. As a society, we have become so enamored with expensive, complicated technologies that we do not trust humble procedures, dating back to ancient times, to possibly work today. The popular thinking seems to say, "If it is not expensive and spectacular, it cannot be any good."

Internal cleansing is too simple.

Testimonial

Depression Diminished

On April 25, I had my first internal cleansing session. I was constipated, overweight, gassy, and for years took three types of anti-depressants. I was never able to get off them. I received fourteen hydrotherapy treatments, and my diet improved. The results were great: more regular BM's, exercising, down to one anti-depressant, clear head, more energy, and I am happier.

Anonymous

Not Out of Gas

An old school chum of mine told me of an incident where she had a "hot" date when she was in her twenties. She was very anxious, as the plan was to go out to dinner to a very elegant restaurant overlooking the ocean.

She dressed up, looking very glamorous. Her date came to the door in his suit, knocked, and then walked her to the car. He opened the door for her, and then proceeded to go around entering the driver's side. As he climbed into the car, he passed gas quite loudly, which destroyed the whole mood of the evening. He said, "Excuse me," but it upset her so much she could not even eat the steak and lobster she ordered at the restaurant. He tried to get a goodnight kiss at the end of the evening, but she could not kiss him. She kept thinking of his gas, which completely repulsed her.

Teenagers usually are embarrassed by internal cleansing, while prepubescent children seem to be good patients.

In today's society, each of us controls our bowels and gas. There is no greater humiliation than publicly having flatulence or soiling oneself. Yet children trained to restrain colon-related opinions can blurt out embarrassing statements.

A client shared she had her date over for a visit. Her niece's five-year-old sat between them, chatting away.

Suddenly, the little girl stopped talking, looked at the man, and in a demanding voice asked, "Did you fart?"

My client was very embarrassed and said, "You should not say that to people!" She then casually commented his breath smelled like flatulence. He had very bad breath.

Toilet Training Attitudes

The root of our reluctance to deal with human elimination and waste is psychological; it has a great deal to do with how we as a society teach our children how and when to eliminate.

Until children are twenty to thirty-six months old, they do not have the completed nerve circuitry to control their sphincters or to connect urinating and bowel movements to being wet or

26

soiled; they do not have the sensations of tightening or relaxing the muscles to pass or hold urine or feces.

During the Victorian era and the Age of Reason, bodily functions were considered necessary evils to the existence of the glorious human mind. They were banned from public notice, at least in the more refined upper strata of society.

Bodily functions were vulgar, common, mean, and unfit for discourse among educated and dignified people. Regimens were enforced, by dictates of betters, but were never mentioned. People ate on schedule, slept on schedule - everything was done according to schedule. People even eliminated on schedule. Naturally, children were reared on a schedule.

Men, the only recognized medical authorities, dictated children must be disciplined and trained into civilized young men and ladies.

Picking up a baby to hold, cuddle, and kiss was discouraged on the grounds it would make the child - especially a boy - a weakling, one who would grow up to be a spineless coward as an adult.

Babies were to begin "potty training" - like puppies - at six months, no later. Even today, some parents boast their children were "potty trained" at nine or ten months.

This early training may have set the stage for our present inability to accept our lower intestine's function and its vital importance.

Urine and feces are not especially disgusting, particularly in a toddler's eyes.

Toddler's go through a normal phase of "discovering" their elimination. One day, usually after a nap, an infant wriggles out of a thoroughly soaked, full diaper, and recognizes in its contents the perfect art medium!

The toddler proceeds to decorate everything in reach, usually his crib and the nearest walls, with this marvelous dark paint.

When Mom opens the nursery door, Junior greets her in ecstatic glee and pride, eager to show off his latest masterpiece. Too bad Mom usually does not appreciate her offspring's budding artistic talent.

Mom's reaction can indicate how she feels about her own body and its functions and how she will introduce her child to the toilet.

If mom feels repulsed and embarrassed about defecation, she will "toilet train" her child, as she was "toilet-trained." She will closely watch her baby for signs he is having a bowel movement; maybe he scrunches up his face and stops what he is doing, or gives some sign.

At the first hint, she will whisk him to the bathroom, where she will plop him on his potty seat, maybe even strapping him in, giving him toys to play with or goodies to eat until he "goes." When he goes, she wipes him, and she may make disgusted faces and comments, maybe even hold her nose, as she hurriedly dumps the feces into the big toilet and flushes them down.

After that trauma, the little one may retain his stool, and become constipated.

When he is finally able to pass his enlarged, hardened feces, they may tear his tender anal tissues. Physical pain and psychological insults will then forever be unconsciously associated with bowel movements.

Testimonial

Elimination dramatically improved

Dear Millan: I am truly amazed at the difference in my eliminating routine.

All my life I have had bowel movements once a week or once every other week. Almost immediately after the first few colon cleansings, I noticed a dramatic change in my eliminating habits. My bowel movements have gone from once a week to once every other day, and sometimes every day.

For me this is truly a miracle. I also had hemor-rhoids that were very painful and would last for days after I had movement.I still have the hemor-rhoids, but because the movements are not hard, the hemorrhoid is far less severe or painful and last only a short time.

I have also changed my diet to fruits, vege-tables and fruit juices. I do eat meat on occasion, but that is very seldom.

I cannot begin to tell you how much better I feel. My dad died from colon cancer and this has always been a great concern of mine.

Colon hydrotherapy has truly been a bless-ing for me.

Joan F.

Using appropriate facilities like adults, chil-dren learn to relieve themselves as needed. They discover that relieving themselves feels good, and they have the right to feel good about it.

Such children have had a positive toilet-learning experience; they learn bowel movements are not only necessary but also good.

I find positively toilet-taught people confide easily and reach a rapid level of trust with their colon hydrotherapist. Psychologists would do well as colon hydrotherapists; they are often clients.

In any case, positive toilet training is more natural. Bowel movements do give relief. They are, after all, waste products and toxic to us.

Bowel movements do not have to be offen-sive. Remember, if we eat healthy foods such as vegetables, fruits, grains, legumes, raw nuts and seeds, and clean out toxins and old matter, our bowel movements will not smell. Nor, if we have the right balance of lactobacilli (friendly flora) and coliform bacilli, will the gas we pass be as offen-sive in odor.

This is great news! We can defecate in any toilet and not be embarrassed.

Sometimes a negatively toilet-trained person can conquer at least some of early conditioning's trauma. Working through past shame, a person can change; personality blocks are overcome. At last, this poor soul will know the benefits of a clean, healthy body. Internal cleanliness is recognized to have tremendous health benefits

Testimonial

No Anal Opening

I was born with an imperferit anus. In other words, there was no anal opening. The lower large intestine was not complete. The doctor performed surgery to create an anal opening. My parents were instructed to hold their fingers in that area so it wouldn't close. My naval protruded and my intestines were pushing against my urinary tract.

I suffered the first years of my life with much pain. I received enemas every day of my life for the first fifteen years. I still became impacted and I had to wear special pants to conceal this problem. I also had no control over my urination.

There was a family friend who was a medical doctor, and he suggested colon hydrotherapy as a last resort before performing the colostomy surgery. The colon hydrotherapist I went to said, "stay on my program for a year and you will be normal." He did not believe my colon was paralyzed as the medical doctors thought. I began with 3 sessions a week, then two a week, then one a week, then one a month over a period of one year. I didn't have to wear special pants any longer, had no more pain, and the urinary tract went back to normal. My bowel movements became normal without enemas. I became a normal, functioning human being, thanks to colon hydrotherapy. Today, I am forty-years-old, and my bowel movements are still normal.

Signed,
Steve

30

The Need for Internal Cleansing

I have been on TV talk shows on numerous occasions discussing internal cleansing and detoxification. Every time, phones ring continuously with people inquiring about internal cleansing. Articles are usually printed in local newspapers: one two-page article was written about me and colon cleansing. After that article appeared, the newspaper received an average of fifty calls a day.

The spread of bubonic plague, and many other diseases, in the Middle Ages was largely due to the personal filthiness of the day. Clean water was eventually discovered to prevent diseases - typhoid fever, cholera, and diarrhea, among others.

Today, the cleaning of skin, teeth, and hair is a basic prerequisite to participating in society.

Not surprisingly, an act of the body so subject to psychological forces holds important implications for health.

One critical balance in the body is between assimilation of nutrients and elimination of the resulting waste products. It seems, however, our homeostatic systems are usually not quite up to peak efficiency. Like all systems, our elimination process is less than one hundred percent efficient.

Therefore, extra dietary bulk and roughage are vital to health. In addition, as washing the skin seems to have a profound, positive effect on health, so too, and even more so, does the washing of the colon.

It seems other cultures and older ways are wiser than we are and could teach us much. It is not so bad to be internally pure.

Take Stock of Attitudes

Take stock of your life: are ingrained attitudes keeping you from living the healthy, vital life you were born to live?

Testimonial

Mental Anguish Gone

Dear Millan:

I am the roommate of Eddie. Prior to his receiving colonics and doing the cleansing program, he would easily get frustrated at the smallest incidence. He would frequently become depressed and angry. I would never know when he would go into a rage and being his roommate was quite challenging.

Since doing the internal cleansing program, Eddie has become a totally different person. Now he doesn't get upset at life's disappointments. He's more mellow, and pleasant to be around. Now what a complete joy having him as a roommate.

Signed, Beverly

2001 Fascinating Facts again states:
In ancient China, doctors [were] paid when their patients were kept well, not when they were sick. Believing that it was the doctor's job to prevent disease. Chinese doctors often paid the patient if the patient lost his health. Further, if a patient died, a special lantern was hung outside the doctor's house. At each death another lantern was added. Too many of these lanterns were certain to ensure a slow trade.

This unique custom would certainly give this country a healthy shaking up! Think of the billions of dollars that would be saved, and the pain and suffering that would be eliminated!

I tell those who want good health to seek out a good, certified colon hydrotherapist and get their whole body cleansed and revitalized! Reward one's struggling body for all its efforts to keep going (despite malnourishing it) by giving it the healthy diet it needs and deserves!

Then, like so many folks who have experienced a detoxification and internal cleansing program, one may boldly, daringly share this experience with someone else. You now know the truth and the truth has set you free.

A middle-aged man came to me for internal cleansing sessions, and when he got to about the fourth cleanse, he began to release large amounts of very old sewage out of the body. He exclaimed, "Why hasn't anyone ever told me about colonics?" I answered with a question. When you leave here, are you going to share with others what has happened to you in the results you have obtained with these cleansing sessions? He stated "hell no". There is your answer.

Another lady did a 10 series of internal cleansings and passed a Barbie doll shoe she had swallowed when she was a little girl.

Testimonial

A Penny Stuck in the Colon

Dear Millan:

I am a model, age twenty-eight, and I began a cleansing program. After my fifth colon cleansing session, I passed a penny. I remember when I was six years old I swallowed that penny; it had been lodged in my colon all these years! The cleansing program flushed it out!

Signed,
Christy

Therapy Could Have Saved Elvis

When Elvis Presley died, the world was shocked. The idol of millions was an unnaturally bloated, unhealthy, and unhappy man. Rumor has it that his autopsy supposedly revealed thirty-two pounds of impacted fecal matter in his colon. Regularly taking many prescription drugs, some incompatible, and suffering evident chronic constipation - caused in part by the medications - caused his untimely and needless death. He died in the bathroom.

I believe, based on countless similar cases, that if Elvis had cleansed his bowels with colon hydrotherapy, gone on a program of a juice fast and cleansing herbs, and then changed his diet, he would be a vigorously alive man today. I also believe his deepening depression may have been caused partly by bad diet and a malfunctioning colon. The prescription drugs were intended to help, but only exacerbated his condition. His doctors tried everything they knew, but Elvis died anyway – trying to have a bowel movement.

CHAPTER FOUR

Quote: Anything worthwhile requires effort. Millan Chessman

CONTROVERSY OF INTERNAL CLEANSING

Internal cleansing is controversial because it deals with the colon, which, as we saw in the previous chapter, is a taboo subject in our society. It is also controversial because it is not supported and is basically ignored by the medical establishment.

Consequently, internal cleansing is regarded as little more than shamanism or bloodletting by leeches according to the medical establishment.

Did you know that the word "leech" is the old Middle English/Anglo-Saxon origin of our word "doctor?" "Leechcraft" is the practice of medicine; "leech" is "doctor!"

The majority of our society is not aware of internal cleansing's existence. The problem is that though no officially recognized research supports this type of therapy, there has been no research that has questioned or condemned it. It languishes in health-care limbo.

Popular thinking goes, "If a medical treatment is not acclaimed in a prestigious medical or research journal, it cannot be good."

Until recently, controversy has muzzled official bans of the procedure. But it seems no one can negate colon hydrotherapy's position.

To bolster their argument against colon hydrotherapy, the medical establishment cites other reports involving rare cases of bowel perforations resulting from incorrectly administered enemas.

These cases were with infants and mental patients in hospitals.

On a few occasions, home enemas, made from fatally toxic mixtures of household cleaners, have been administered by overzealous parents to their constipated or ill children. Of these cases, some resulted in water-intoxication and death.

This sad reliance on exceptional and irrelevant examples demonstrates the depth of the medical establishment's ignorance, even among specialists in the fields of gastroenterology and oncology.

Among practitioners of western medicine, internal cleansing remains misunderstood. In the first place, distinctions between colon hydrotherapy and enema usage are fuzzy. In the second place, internal cleansing's practical therapeutic applications go unrecognized, and state-of-the-art procedures and equipment go under-utilized.

Few schools offer the necessary detailed training and internships. This is largely a result of the medical establishment's stubborn refusal to accept internal cleansing; therefore, the American Medical Association will not recognize it, let alone establish standardized curriculums at accredited professional teaching and training facilities. A person who cuts hair must be licensed in all states except Florida, yet a colon hydrotherapist is yet to be licensed in California as of this writing.

Ongoing Debate

Among medical professionals in the last seventy years, internal cleansing's popularity has declined until recently. Misconceptions about the physiology and the efficacy of the colon resulted in wrong advice. For instance, some believe that two or three correctly administered colon therapies would sufficiently cleanse the body.

Today, we know this is not true. Unfortunately, this bogus perception contributed to the medical profession's dismissing internal cleansing as ineffective.

Medical practitioners seem to be either whole-heartedly in favor of or adamantly against modern internal cleansing.

Those in favor are usually those who have benefited from it or have been open-minded. Skeptics are almost always those who have no such knowledge or experience.

I heard a pastor once say, "Prejudice is when you are down on something you are not up on."

Tracking the Progress of Internal cleansing Through the Medical Literature

During the 1930's colon irrigation was regularly reviewed in the *New England Journal of Medicine, The British Medical Journal,* and *Lancet.* A comprehensive work was compiled by W. Kerr Russell, MD, assistant editor of the *British Journal of Physical Medicine* in 1932.

Several books published since 1981 by gastroenterologists refer to "the end of the colonic era" around 1960. Since 1960, ignorance, misinformation, and failure by the AMA to recognize internal cleansing's legitimacy have prevented standard medical doctors from prescribing the procedure. Consequently, within the medical establishment, prejudices surround the subject.

There is an unwillingness to examine the actual results of internal cleansing.

Throughout the 1980's, many bowel-related books were written. Their medical authors describe various bowel diseases, possible causes, and corrective surgical procedures. Some of these recent books approach better bowel health through diet. Some even mention enemas and colema boards.

Unfortunately, many discourage colon hydrotherapy - if they mention it at all - on purely unfounded facts. So many of them have not researched the subject, interviewed practitioners or patients involved in internal cleansing, or received treatment themselves.

37

In United States history, millions of people have had colon hydrotherapy.

Legitimate criticisms of techniques and lack of sanitation while giving enemas can be found, but since the 1930's there has been no published scientific literature disclaiming the effectiveness of colon hydrotherapy.

An article in *The Journal of Joint and Manipulative Therapy* once mistakenly criticized colon hydrotherapy and enemas for removing all the bacteria from the lower GI tract. These critics seemed ignorant of the fact that most colon hydrotherapy is directed at removing poisons and restoring normal colon function.

Inclusive Approach to Health

Not too long ago, doctors sneered at the thought of healing herbs. Yet progress is being made in the established medical profession, and change is being implemented in medical philosophy and attitudes, toward a more inclusive approach to health.

As recently as the early 1980's, the medical professionals' official position was, "heart disease is linked to a bad diet." Prior to that they scoffed at the idea diet could affect the condition of the heart. Anyone who claimed otherwise was a quack, a far-out, fringe crackpot, and a counterfeit.

A Case of Misdiagnosis

My friend Ken told me of a time when he was twelve. He did not want to go to school and so told his mother that he was sick. She let him stay home.

The next day he told her he was sick again. She let him stay home again. The third day he told her he was sick again.

She said, "Well, then, it is time to take you to the doctor." At the clinic, the doctor asked him, "Where does it hurt?" Ken stated, "Here," and pointed to his right side, exactly where the appendix was.

The doctor ran some extensive tests and afterwards announced, "This boy is having an appendicitis attack! We need to get him to a hospital immediately for surgery."

His mother was horrified and felt remorse for not taking her child to the doctor sooner. Of course, she consented, and he was rushed to the hospital for an appendectomy.

Thirty-five years later he was visiting his mother and announced, "Mom, remember when I had my appendix taken out? Well, I want to tell you I never had any pain on my side, and was never sick. I just did not want to go to school." Ken's mother was shocked.

When Ken's doctor examined that appendix, he undoubtedly knew it did not warrant removal, and probably knew that before and when he made his diagnosis.

What a barbaric thing to do to a human being, especially a child!

Testimonial

How Internal cleansing Brought Financial Success

About two years ago, I received a telephone call from a client:

Hello, Millan.

I do not know if you remember me. My name is Glen, and I did an internal cleansing program from you a year ago.

I am a traveling salesman, and at that time my health was a mess. I was desperate because my sales quota was very low and my livelihood was at stake. I had absolutely no energy or enthusiasm. I am here to tell you, one year after those treatments, I have made a million dollars in sales! Millan, it is all thanks to your help and your program.

Thank you!   *Anonymous*

Unnatural Treatment?

Another objection from the establishment to internal cleansing is that the procedure is "unnatural." Yet, even in our natural state, we, as human beings, are, of all Nature's creatures, wholly unnatural.

Cooking food - whether over a fire, in an oven, a microwave, on a stovetop, is not natural. Surgery is unnatural.

The most unnatural thing that people do these days is eat unnatural foods: foods that have all the good fiber processed out; foods in which enzymes necessary for vitamin and mineral assimilation are destroyed through cooking; flesh foods; pasteurized and homogenized dairy products; foods that have harmful hormones, chemicals, dyes, additives, preservatives, pesticides, and chemical fertilizers.

Supposedly, the medical community considers our diet to be wholly and completely natural for human beings.

Get the picture?

That medical doctors can even protest unorthodox therapeutic practices such as colon hydrotherapy is an oxymoron.

Thus, the pseudo-argument against the "unnaturalness" of internal cleansing falls apart. The people performing the most unnatural of procedures - pouring and popping unnatural chemicals, in the form of syrups and pills, down the throats of unwell patients; cutting people open and rearranging or removing internal body parts; making surgical patients sleep an unnatural sleep under unnatural and dangerous chemical anesthesia - are those protesting that internal cleansing is "unnatural." All this because internal cleansing simply and gently puts warm sanitized water into and out of human colons.

Does that make sense? There is something very wrong here.

Many opponents of internal cleansing object to it as being "unnatural." Yes, it is unnatural to

40

put water in the colon, but eating the diet we do, of foods laced with man-made chemical pesticides, herbicides, hormones, and preservatives, is most unnatural!

Our bodies were never designed to take in foods with chemicals, dyes, pesticides, synthetic hormones, preservatives, and all the rest. When we eat processed, overcooked foods, our bodies cannot digest and break down nutrients for proper assimilation.

Man-made foods do us harm in many ways, still not fully understood by science. And if the scientific community still does not comprehend the full impact of certain food substances on the human body, do not think the makers and licensees of additives and enhancers do either! This is how we get into health trouble.

What is Natural

A prescription may or may not help the sufferer; often it adds new problems. But someone who does internal cleansing enjoys improved health almost immediately. And the new lease on life is accomplished without dangerous, unknown side effects, or allergic reactions.

What is natural for us is to return to a clean, healthy, and efficient colon sustained by a healthful diet.

As with any naturally positive process, one must start by getting rid of what is wrong and then doing what is right.

The immediate response from an ailing colon to a cleansing session is very positive. In its own quiet way, a newly rejuvenated colon is the answer to all objections that internal cleansing is "unnatural."

Again, I will say it, "In order to regain health, one must start by getting rid of what is wrong and then do what is right."

Internal cleansing helps do exactly that.

Without drugs, anesthesia, knives, radiation, or chemotherapy, internal cleansing and detoxification are preemptive steps against disease, with no added harm to the body.

Testimonial

A Case of Restored Fertility

Believe it or not, even some conditions of infertility can be an effect of an unhealthy colon, as Sherry, a client, illustrates:

For five years, my husband and I tried very hard to have a baby but could not. I was artificially inseminated many times. I developed a cyst in the ovaries from the side effects of the medication I had to take.
Finally, my husband and I had internal cleansing in a series of ten-colon cleansings for each of us.
We also followed the cleansing program Millan recommended.
One month after we completed our series, I got pregnant.
I honestly believe cleansing our bodies and strengthening our immune systems had something to do with my getting pregnant.
Since going through the cleansing program, my cyst is gone and we now have a beautiful healthy baby boy!

Sherry

Testing the Wrong Option: A Study of Hyperactive Children

A recent study tested two groups of hyperactive children. One group was fed a concentrated sugar diet. The other group was given food sweetened with cyclamates and saccharin. Neither the children nor their parents knew what the children were eating. The parents kept records of their children's behavior.

The study found that "the children acted the same on either one of these sweeteners."

42

Final conclusion: there was no difference in either group's behavior.

What a shame!

Why not take one group of these children off all the chemical-filled junk and put them on natural, God-made foods such as fresh fruits and vegetables? Then there would surely be a difference.

Regrettably, individual families that I know of have already proven these findings. The parents in this study simply removed one bad thing from their children and replaced it with another.

It frustrates me to see these kinds of studies conducted, especially since you and I probably paid for that study with our hard-earned tax dollars. Now, no doubt, the families with hyperactive children will continue to let them eat all of the sugary foods they want, never knowing the real answer.

Electrolyte Depletion?

It is argued that colon hydrotherapy sessions can deplete a patient's electrolytes.

Electrolytes are vital to health and life, and are instantly replaced by eating. A good suggestion would be to drink a glass of whole, natural fruit juice.

Testimonial

More Energy Now

Dear Millan:
I was attending a breast cancer night at SK sanctuary. The consultant and I continued to share information and stories about health. Never did I know that this conversation would change my life forever. She started telling me about her mother Millan and the importance of internal cleansing. I told her that I was diagnosed with breast cancer and had a simple lumpectomy followed with radiation. Later I was diagnosed with colon cancer. I couldn't believe that this was happening to me

43

once again. This surgery was not so simple this time and my recovery took a while.

I have always had good health and practiced some alternative medicine, so to become ill was very hard for me. I really felt like my body had failed me; however, I had failed my body.

I maintained a good diet consisting of the "Pyramid Food Group," which I now believe is not such a good diet and that it did attribute to my poor health.

I was so grateful to have met Millan and couldn't absorb enough information that she had to give me. It was like an answer to my prayers. Millan, you have given me so much insight on diet, body, health, and spirituality.

The cleansing and diet changes have given me more energy than I thought possible. I only wish I knew about internal cleansing years ago. I really believe I could have avoided my illnesses.

I have informed all my family and highly recommend internal cleansing for everyone, especially before the body becomes ill with disease.

Fondly in His love,
Dottie E.

Nutritional Controversies

The following statements were made on a televised report on health; with news anchor Jim Wilkerson reporting. Various medical experts gave their opinions as to current health information.

Earl Mendell, vitamin author, states:

Doctors state that we need milk for strong bones. Really?

Five studies show that the five leading nations consuming the most milk daily have the highest incidence of osteoporosis, while nations consuming no dairy products have no osteoporosis.

In recent years, the agriculture department has announced a new shape for the ideal diet. Instead of the familiar pie chart of the

44

so-called basic food groups, the new shape is a pyramid emphasizing grains and not much fat.

It is no wonder there is so much confusion. It is said that only a third of the medical schools require students to study nutrition. Courses in preventive medicine, nutrition and exercise are seldom taught in our nation's medical schools. Instead, medical students are subjected to course after course on pharmacology. They are taught that drugs are the more useful tools for treating disease.

No one wants to tell Americans they are lazy and set in their ways, or that they cry too easily to doctors when they get sick, leaving an unpayable $800 billion medical bill. On the one hand, people cry because no one takes care of them, and, on the other hand, they are not willing themselves to prevent disease.

People must take charge of their own health.

Mendell also states, *"We spend 97% of our health care dollars on sickness and only 3% on prevention."*

On the same broadcast, Dr. Gary Knoll, author and medical reporter, states, *"We are the sickest nation in the world. We have the highest medical bill in the world. We eat the worst food in the world and yet we have the best food in the world, we're just not eating it."*

News anchor Jim Wilkerson reported:

"The purest foods are available in the health food stores, and the government strangles them by considering legislation that would make vitamins and herbs prescription only. So, we're looking at the safest industry in the free world, the industry of nutritional supplements, yet the FDA wants to regulate that industry out of existence. It is the safest industry we have. It is totally insane.

It is time we take control of our own bodies!

45

A recent cover story of Time magazine told how new research has shown that vitamins may help fight cancer, heart disease, and aging. The article claimed, "Only 9% of the American people eat well enough to get all their nutrients from foods." I called the FDA in Washington and got phone bounced four times until, finally, I got to a guy who would take my questions about chelation, tryptophane, and about the health food industry, and he said he would mail me a position paper that very day. And that was more than two weeks ago. I haven't received a thing.

Prevention is of primary importance.

In a news story regarding health, Dr. Gary Knoll states:

The basic four-food groups concept is a fraud, an absolute fraud. It is voodoo science, it is witchcraft, and it is the worst abomination. It's what's killing us. We have the most tyrannical bureaucracy in the world in the form of the FDA. There is no limit on alcohol or tobacco we can put into our body, but they want to cut back on the amount of nutrients we can have that can be prevention.

Julian Wittacher, M.D., states, *"Bypass surgery, for instance, has failed miserably."* He cites two government-funded, controlled studies to establish long-term benefits of prevention, and he showed supported studies from the AMA.

"In the list of facts doctors cannot tell their patients, but want them to know, doctors are terrified of two things: 'malpractice suits and being labeled non-conformist.'

The doctors' job is not to keep them well, but to help them after they get sick. The more costly the procedure, tests and drugs, the more the system makes. The crisis intervention of medicine and the use of aggressive therapies in many cases when they are not warranted are bankrupting the country."

Dr. Wittacher has investigated the medical profession for twenty years and has written dozens of books. He writes:

I worked with Dr. Pritigen back in 1976, and I saw large numbers of people get well. Yet, when I was in medical school and medical training, I never saw anybody get well. I saw people get better. I saw people get out of the hospital with their prescription, and many came back, and we never really learn how to make people well. I think that it is time that the American public realizes the FDA is not necessarily looking out for your best interest. They're on their own, because no one in the American system has the guts to say to the American people 'Change or die.'

Earl Mendell, on Channel 10 News, states:

The government had outlawed tryptophan. Some people died after taking the popular natural sleep inducing amino acid. But investigation proved it was a tainted batch from Japan, but tryptophan was still banned.

I think it was working too well, and I think it was starting to hurt the sale of other drugs. It's interesting that they had a tainted Tylenol. In two days, it is back on the market.

Hooked on Colonics?

Another protest from ignorant but vocal medical personnel is that internal cleansing can be "addictive" or habit-forming. There has not been one case I know of where a person cannot have a bowel movement without a colonic.

Just the opposite is true.

Those with severe constipation are inversely helped in overcoming this condition.

The other dependency cited as a possibility is based on a primary misunderstanding of what internal cleansing actually is.

Most opponents fuzzily equate internal cleansing with a laxative.

This assumption is erroneous!

Laxatives use chemicals that irritate the lining of the colon, making it convulse defensively. When laxatives are used too much, the natural peristalsis of the colon, weakened by constipation to begin with, desists entirely, and the body must then wait for the laxative to stimulate contraction of the colon's muscles. In time, increasing amounts of the laxative are required to obtain the desired result. This condition is dangerous for obvious reasons, and is in reality a chemical dependence.

There are about three hundred varieties of laxatives. They are the number two drug sold in the U.S.A.

I would say this country has an uptight anus!

How Many Sessions?
In interviews with doctors and health practitioners regarding internal cleansing, I was surprised to hear many say that people need only three sessions of colon hydrotherapy.

The reasons given were:

1.) "Too much colon-cleansing can be habit-forming."

2.) "People become dependent upon colon-cleansings like they do laxatives."

3.) "You will detox and cleanse the colon completely with three treatments."

Nothing can be further from the truth. On the contrary, the reverse happens.

I stated earlier that the colon is a muscular organ often impacted with stool. When the colon is unburdened and exercised, it works more efficiently. I have seen this happen repeatedly.

My question to one doctor was, "Have you ever seen any instances of colon hydrotherapy becoming habit-forming and the bowel not being able to evacuate as a result?"

His answer was, "No."

48

He had only given his opinion without providing any facts.

My thirty plus years in the field of detox/fasting and internal cleansing has shown that to thoroughly detoxify and cleanse the colon, a minimum of ten treatments is necessary.

Costly Colostomies

Indications are that the practice of surgical colostomies is more profitable than referring patients to colon hydrotherapists.

If a doctor cannot get a patient's colon to work properly after inundating it with drugs, laxatives, and an exam performed by a nurse, a colostomy is performed. In this surgery, the colon is surgically removed and replaced with a tube at the end of the small intestine. This tube is connected to a plastic bag worn outside the body.

The patient loses out under the knife, and gains endless embarrassment as bags have leaked, stunk, and often collapsed during changing. In addition, complications can arise, and ongoing medical and prescription bills and wrangling with reluctant insurance companies provide a constant headache.

Not a pretty picture!

One colostomy recipient went for a job interview. Somehow, his bag broke and the stool spilled on the prospective employer's office floor. That applicant was so humiliated he went and committed suicide.

Someone very dear to me had a colostomy, and when I visited him I could hear the gas pass into his bag. He had no control over this. This was very humiliating to this honorable man.

How sad and yet unnecessary.

Contrasting this lengthy and costly procedure, internal cleansing improves the health of clients to the point where they actually do not need to visit the doctor.

Ultimate Goal of Internal Cleansing

Basically, the colon is like an old water pipe. It keeps getting more sluggish and flaccid from daily ingestion of the wrong foods.

We take better care of our cars than we do our bodies.

We change the oil and lubricate our autos at the recommended times because we want our cars to last longer and run better, without expense later.

I believe our bodies and brains are like the engines in our cars. There are either four, six, or eight cylinders, but if operating on only two, the performance will be poor.

However, how often do we clean out the digestive system where sewage lies stagnating?

How can we expect to live long, healthy, and energetic lives if we do not clean out the build-up put in by destructive living habits?

In contrast to laxatives, colon hydrotherapy "jump-starts" a sluggish colon into renewed peristaltic vigor!

Over time, an unresponsive colon is stimulated into natural peristaltic action by the gentle introduction and evacuation of water, cleansing of its clogged passageway. Normal peristaltic action to eliminate a normal waste load can be reestablished. Since colon hydrotherapy uses only filtered water, - no drugs - no type of chemical dependency can develop.

After cleaning out the overburdened, constipated, or non-functioning colon, the natural peristalsis is restored; the colon can now resume normal operation on its own, unassisted. This is why we call it colon hydrotherapy; doing therapy on the colon.

This, in fact, is the ultimate goal of internal cleansing and that is washing out waste, resulting in detoxifying the body.

Sleep Improved

Dearest Millan,

    I am totally impressed!! The love and compassion I felt while under your care was wonderfully refreshing. I walked out of your office with a bounce in my step and a renewed joy in my heart. I felt so wonderfully relaxed that even the heavy traffic nor the stupid drivers could upset me on the way home. I haven't slept so well in months. I woke with such vigor that I accomplished on Saturday what I wanted to do for months and even years. The last three months have been a new awakening of my life. I turned 49 years in August and I suddenly realized that I couldn't continue to abuse my body if I wish to live a long and healthy life and see my grandchild grow. He was born last January and he is the real joy of my life.

    I was drinking a case of beer and nearly three packs of cigarettes a day and I felt terrible. Nothing gave me satisfaction. I would drink from the time I awoke until I fell asleep, which even sleep became difficult. I was lucky if I got 4 or 5 hours. I always felt tense and the anxiety was totally unbelievable. I couldn't eat because my stomach felt like it was tied in knots. The depression became so intense at times that I seriously considered suicide!

    I began to rationalize my existence and realized that what I had been doing to my body and mind was no longer acceptable. I began to look to the medical profession for help and boy was that a disaster. All I got was a lot of "I don't know" and a long row of pill bottles. After weeks of this disgusting scenario, I realized that only I could help myself. I began to open my eyes to the things and people around me who I previously had a closed mind about. I began to attend church with my sister and nieces and really feel wonderful that I now have the Lord in my heart. With this new awakening, each day brings with it new surprises and new feelings. I have had a motto clipped onto my refrigerator door for years. It never really had the meaning that it has now. It says: THIS IS THE FIRST DAY OF THE REST OF YOUR LIFE. DON'T BLOW IT! I realize now that the word that best describes my past life is "indifference." Indifferent to friends who practice a wholistic and healthy lifestyle; indifferent to family members who believe that having the Lord in your life will bring unbelievable happiness. And now I have found you. I seriously feel that the Lord has led me to you. The aura I felt from the moment I entered your office was unique and unlike anything I've experienced before. The openness and compassion was wonderful. I must admit I was very nervous when I entered your office.

This was a totally different experience and I must admit that I feared it would be a painful experience. Those fears were totally unfounded. You explained fully each step of the way. It was the most painless and eye opening experience I have ever had, unlike experiences with the medical profession. It was much less painful than giving myself an enema. I was totally amazed at how much waste came out of my body during the cleanse session.

Your book is wonderful and I must admit that I couldn't put it down and am now re-reading it. I look forward to a lifelong relationship with you.

With love and compassion for what you have done for my health.

Thank you,
Robert

CHAPTER FIVE

Quote: Defeat is a blessing in disguise, to get one step closer to victory and success. Millan Chessman

MEDICAL PROFESSION

A Changing Health Field

Modern medicine has remarkably low cure rates for the diseases and conditions it treats. Dissatisfied patients are seeking more effective and less expensive answers to their physical ailments. Alternatives to costly procedures offer more wholistic approaches to wellness.

Testimonial

My Breathing Has Improved

One client wrote me:

My father died suddenly in bed three weeks before his ninety-ninth birthday. He was very active and had many colon cleansing sessions during his lifetime.

Years ago, I had a few colon cleansing sessions and then forgot about them until recently. A friend told me about her colon hydrotherapist and what the therapy had done for her. I am sure our Lord worked this out to help me regain better health.

I have had several sessions, and now I truly have a new lease on life.

Three years ago, I was put on oxygen eighteen hours a day because I have chronic obstructive pulmonary disease (COPD). I was married for 26 years to a smoker, although I never smoked. I have been diagnosed with asthma and emphysema as a result of the second-hand smoke.

About four months ago, I broke my left shoulder. Since then, to help me breathe, I have increased my dose of Ventolyn Spray medication to every three hours.

Every four hours is the maximum dosage. However, since my cleanse, my breathing has improved. This past week I have gone four, five, and even six hours between Ventolyn doses. It is truly wonderful to sleep six hours without interruption.

My energy level increases daily, and I feel so much more alive. The junk and toxins shed during my colon cleansing sessions reveal why I have not been in good health. It is unbelievable all that was in my intestines - undoubtedly for many years - since I was constipated a good part of my life.

Anyone who has ever been constipated would greatly benefit from internal cleansing. Some people believe it can add ten years to your life, and I concur heartily.

Signed,
Dorothy M.

AMA - Internal Cleansing's Challenge

The challenge a colon hydrotherapist faces is at least threefold:

First, there is resistance from the AMA. Clients have stated internal cleansing provides both immediate health and longevity.

The practical evidence is abundant, yet the AMA requires repeatable results from standardized tests. Interestingly, such tests have never been conducted.

Without documented experimental and clinical results and thorough studies, the evidence for internal cleansing cannot be discredited.

The AMA may be revealing the medical industry's interest in maintaining the lucrative status quo of ill health; it is well known that some doctors maintain their high standards of living at the expense of unnecessary and unhealthy conditions of their dependent patients.

A healthy person means lost revenues for the medical establishment. Increased health means a lower demand for high-cost, high-tech "medicine."

Internal cleansing is low-cost and low-tech. It can be administered by someone other than a fully licensed medical doctor, but we must no longer deny its effectiveness.

Second, I believe internal cleansing should be a standard office procedure with medical doctors, chiropractors, naturopaths and acupuncturists.

Third, and perhaps most important, is the challenge to people themselves. People need to take control of their bodies.

Someone else's scare tactics should not influence our health decisions. We should find health professionals who offer workable procedures. Time is too short to waste on treatments that do nothing but bring disease, suffering, and even premature death.

A.M.A. Forced to Cover Backside

In recent decades the medical community has provided several examples of wrong thinking. For example, until the late 1970's, despite studies that clearly showed otherwise, the medical establishment denied any connection between heart disease, diet, and exercise. In the early 1980's, the public demanded an accounting, but instead of acknowledging the error, the A.M.A. simply issued its own authoritative guidelines for heart health.

A.M.A. and the doctors implied as if they themselves had known and practiced the new approach all along!

A similar tactic was used on the issue of high blood pressure; that battle for patient participation and self-care is still ongoing.

In the sixties, a TV comedy sketch depicted a scene in which a patient (a smoker), hacking and coughing miserably, goes to see his doctor. The doctor has him sit on the examining table, and, with ear to stethoscope, has the patient take a deep breath.

As he does so, the doctor, himself smoking an extra long cigarette, goes into a lengthy spasm of coughing. The patient takes the stethoscope out of the doctor's limp hand and has the doctor sit up on the examining table; whereupon, the patient proceeds to listen to the doctor's chest and recommends that the physician quit smoking!

Until the Surgeon General's announcement that smoking unequivocally causes cancer and emphysema, doctors were actually touting health benefits of smoking!

Ironically, doctors maintain that they are on the side of freedom of choice. These are the same doctors who would deny colon hydrotherapists the right to perform a procedure with NO deleterious health effects, a method of treatment, which is, by all indications, a vital tool in promoting optimal health, as a FREE CHOICE to their patients.

FDA's Opposition
Health-food stores are doing their best business ever! More and more people are beginning to recognize the benefits of organic vegetables, fruits, and over-the-counter herbs.

For years, the Food and Drug Administration (FDA) has kept a watchful eye on the sale of herbs and vitamins.

The FDA claims vitamins and herbs must be regulated to ensure public safety. FDA opponents believe regulation is just another way for those in the medical field to maintain control of the vitamin industry and its profits.

Many observers believe the AMA is attempting to control alternative forms of treatment. More and more, patients are gravitating to workable methods of staying healthy, and not just treating symptoms.

Proponents of colon hydrotherapy have advocated controlled research studies initiated by the medical establishment, but to no avail. These studies would help convince the medical community that colon hydrotherapy is safe and effective. They would also bring colon hydrotherapy into the mainstream of modern medicine and bring it to the public's eye. Research would also vindicate the many patients who, over the decades have benefited physically, medically and psychologically from internal cleansing.

Harassment of a Colon Hydrotherapist

The following account is from a letter written to me by a Colon Hydrotherapist living in San Francisco who was arrested for simply performing colon hydrotherapy:

Not too long ago, in February, an undercover person who identified herself as Janine Flannery called to make an appointment for colon hydrotherapy. She came to my office the following week. She filled out my intake sheet and took the procedure as far as putting on the gown I offered her. At this point, she just stalled by talking and asking questions like, 'What was this going to do to her?' and 'How does this equipment work?' She made me nervous! I suggested some books to read to give her additional information in helping her decide if this was in fact what she really wanted to do. We had spent the better part of 45 minutes at this point. Although she didn't follow through on the actual colon hydrotherapy, she paid me as though she had tak-

57

en the colonic, requesting a receipt for ser-
vices rendered, and I in return supplied her
with one, as well as two leaflets copied from a
book which they later used in court to show
intent to commit the violation and to make a
case around it.

Upon her departure, a sense of fear envel-
oped me. Within 5 minutes, a persistent
knocking and ringing of the doorbell ensued.
I would not answer the door. I walked to the
window and to my astonishment; I watched
her ride away with a man I recognized as the
Senior Investigator of the AMA. Anxiety
stricken, I was comfortable that I had said
nor done NOTHING incriminating! Later, I
found out she was wired for sound.

On April 1, a client walked into my office
at 9 a.m. Three minutes later, there was a
knocking at my door. I didn't answer because
I was expecting my client only. The knocking
became a relentless banging, which in turn
greatly upset my client. I reluctantly opened
the door, and was faced with an impeccably
dressed couple - a male and a female. I was
greeted with, 'Are you Delores Hepburn?' and
I replied, 'Yes, I am.' The female flashed her
badge and identified the two of them. She
said, 'You are under arrest.' I asked for her
warrant. She grabbed my wrist and pulled
me through the door onto my porch. She said,
'Don't make trouble.' I asked to get a purse
and coat and was denied. One of them closed
my door, locking my client in and me out
with no keys or money. I was asked to face the
wall. Then they handcuffed my arms behind
me. At this moment, I felt embarrassment for
what my neighbors might wonder about me.
Did she murder someone? I was directed to a
waiting car 100 yards up the street. I walked
in handcuffs with the officers behind me - my
head down. I did not want to see a neighbor
looking at me in this position.

When we arrived at the police station, I was asked to give fingerprints and let them take my picture. I refused, as it is my constitutional right to do so. I am not a criminal - I had done nothing wrong. I simply administered colon hydrotherapy. I was threatened with stripping me of all my clothes and being thrown into 'the hole' if I did not submit to a full set of fingerprints.

When the officers in the station were angry enough, one of them twisted my arm up behind my back and cuffed me again. At this point, they put ink on my fingers and pressed paper to them. I was taken to a day room where I was further intimidated by drug addicts, prostitutes and other people displaying bruises on their faces inflicted by the police (according to them). I didn't speak the language of anyone in there. I felt sheer terror! I was told by a day officer, 'People in jail have no rights except to be fed and have a place to sleep.' At this time, I was informed that I would have to sleep on the floor without a blanket or a mat. The thought of sleeping on concrete and the fact that I had a foster child coming home from camp the next day quickly prompted me to do what I had to do to leave that awful place.

I let them take my picture and gave them a complete set of fingerprints. I signed my name under duress and walked away a free person as long as I showed up for court the next day. However, I still didn't have a coat nor did I have a quarter to make a phone call. I walked from the police station to the Salvation Army; from there I made a call to a friend who came to pick me up. As I waited, I reflected on what had happened to me. I felt raped multiple times. Stripped of all my dignity and any self worth I ever had. Helpless and homeless because a locksmith was not going to get me into my house for free.

*The court was not always kind to me be-
cause I was my own representative. After every hearing, the District Attorney badgered me
with 'You can't win your case. Give up and
take the alternative program.' In essence,
their proposal of an alternative program was
an admission of guilt further penalized by
community service projects. Where was the
law I had broken? On June 12, my case was
dismissed, bringing to a close 21 months and
11 days of emotional hell! If I was subjected
to this kind of treatment without there being
a law against the subject matter, what would
happen if there was one? I am not a criminal,
and have never broken any laws. I don't know
what the future holds for me. Three years
have gone by. I did not escape damage. My
heart beats rapidly whenever someone knocks
on my door, or stranger parks near my home.*

*My enthusiasm and warmth I was once
able to impart to each person I met is suppressed. Everyone who calls me is suspect. I
am no longer comfortable to be my naturally
energetic, animated self. I love working with
people and helping them to become healthy.
There is strength in numbers. I hope that in
the future there will be many voices speaking
out collectively to defend our right to continue
this work. I am grateful to have had the opportunity to grow by way of standing up for
something I believe in.*

Delores Hepburn

Pharmaceuticals

Because of new products from burgeoning pharmaceutical companies, doctors began to discount
colon cleansing as a legitimate and valuable medical practice.

In the 1920's, John D. Rockefeller invested
millions of dollars in certain pharmaceutical companies and bought out some prestigious but floun-

dering medical schools. Consequently, doctors learned to write out prescriptions, which the pharmaceutical companies filled with their products. As a result, current drugs and technology have all but replaced simple, natural, preventive health practices.

Until the 1970's, chiropractic clinics offering colon cleansing existed nationwide. Now, only a few remain. This is unfortunate, since adjustments stay longer when internal cleansing is included.

The decline in medically prescribed colon hydrotherapy has spurred an increase of independent colon hydrotherapists. These service an informed and often desperate public. Seeking relief, patients feel their doctors cannot alleviate ill conditions they may have.

Did you know?
San Diego County sewer plant gathers and removes five 55-gallon drums of vitamins, pills and tablets per day.

Testimonial

A Relieved Client

I was a mess health-wise. First, I have been constipated and have suffered terrible gas all my life. Second, I have had hemorrhoids since childhood. Inexplicably, another serious problem developed regular bouts of vomiting. Despite numerous tests, doctors were unable to help me.

I then started internal cleansing with Millan. She put me on a detoxifying diet of herbs, and I did a series of twelve-colon hydrotherapy sessions.

My life changed: my bowels moved more regularly, my gas problem disappeared, my energy level increased, and I started exercising regularly and drinking a lot of water.

My hemorrhoids were not as uncomfortable as before, and my vomiting stopped.

Signed,
Juanita

Pill Therapy vs. Internal Cleansing

Some fear unknown side effects from internal cleansing. To many, as we saw in Chapter Three, discussions of body elimination can be repulsive. This may be one reason why pill therapy this century has been so embraced by doctors and their patients alike.

The solution pills offer seems simple, neat, and fast acting. However, pill therapy falls short of the mark. While in many cases the main effect of prescription drugs seems nothing short of miraculous, many drugs carry side effects that may turn out to be more devastating than the symptoms they were intended to treat. In addition, pill therapy leaves the body in a toxic state. Remember, pills treat the symptoms, not the cause.

Despite this knowledge, doctors continue to prescribe medications. They may or may not briefly discuss possible side effects with the patient, but gloss over negative possibilities to alleviate patient anxiety. For, in terms of time and effort, it inconveniences a doctor when a patient balks at taking medication and takes the doctor's valuable time to inquire about all the information regarding the prescription.

Beware of Drugs' Side Effects

Side effects should not be overlooked.

Indeed, when you get a prescription, usually enclosed is a tightly folded page listing the drug's "contraindications." The text is in such tiny print you may legitimately wonder if you were intended to read it. These "contraindications" are known side effects associated with the medication. The literature details their seriousness, the conditions under which they occur, and results of related experiments. The wording is dry and clinical, often unintelligible to the lay reader, so as not to arouse alarm.

Doctors may expect patients to take medication on an ongoing basis, not knowing if patients will show recognized symptoms of side effects or how particular bodies will react to certain drugs.

In the event a patient reacts negatively, the doctor will make one of two choices: to adjust the dosage and see what happens, or discontinue that drug and try another one. Even after all the clinical testing of a drug, the patient is still a guinea pig, because everyone's body differs in its chemical interactions.

Ironically, the same doctors who prescribe drugs with known deleterious side effects caution against internal cleansing because of its possible "unknown" side effects!

This, despite there being absolutely NONE on record anywhere. Again, these doctors try to hide behind an old smokescreen. They maintain there are no "scientific, peer-reviewed" studies to document the safety of internal cleansing.

Testimonial

Zoloft and A Negative Attitude

Dear Millan:

Thanks for the help. The time spent with you, and the colonics I received, have been like a breath of fresh air.

Before knowing you, I was on Zoloft pills (100 mg) and had a very negative attitude towards life and myself, not to mention the way I smelled. My body was so out of tune that I was like a mummy. I was very tired all of the time. Now, spiritually, everyday is my birthday after each colonic session.

Since I am a June baby, the sun is back to shine on

> *me. Thank you so much for helping to bring back my true*
> *colors. The real Larry C. can now stand up.*
> *Sincerely,*
> *Larry C.*

Clearly, the medical establishment is not about to begin a study! Who knows what acute or long-term damage is taking place while many are taking prescription drugs? And these medications may lead to complications that have no corrective recourse.

An example of just such a complication is a condition known as "dry mouth," which occurs as a side effect of over four hundred prescription drugs. It is usually discovered by dentists attempting to treat patients complaining of this symptom. Because the salivary glands fail to secrete enough saliva (which contains digestive enzymes that kill many harmful bacteria, thus keeping the enamel-eating bacteria neutralized), patients tend to experience an increase in the number of dental cavities.

Reluctant M.D.'s
For the present, people just do not want to discuss the colon. Even a number of medical doctors do not really want to neither talk about it nor listen to patients' complaints about it.

People may find they complain to their M.D.'s of constipation. Their doctors will immediately write a prescription for a laxative, and that would be the last of that subject.

M.D.'s seldom involving themselves with what they feel is an offensive part of the body. Too few seem to recognize the importance of a clean colon. Many find the topic just as offensive as their patients do, having in common conditioning by society. But with enough people learning and experiencing the extraordinary health benefits of this important therapy, this can change. Become one of these people!

Testimonial

Fasting Lowered Fat and Sugar Levels

Before I came to Millan for a fasting and colon cleansing program, my triglycerides and cholesterol level were high, and I was concerned. I fasted on the juices and did the colon cleansing sessions each day for seven days. I then went back to the doctor and was tested; my levels were down to normal! I feel great, and my belly went flat!

Signed,
Ron

A Doctor's Orders

Once, a medical doctor referred a cancer patient to me. The man was suffering from constipation, which was caused by medications he was taking to combat his disease. He was, unfortunately, in the last stages of this illness.

Gently, I gave him colon hydrotherapy, which washed out some of the impacted matter from his lower colon. He felt slight relief, and, as he was to return home back east the next day, I bade him good-bye, thinking I would probably never hear from him again.

His colon's arrested peristalsis had been stimulated by the cleansing and was trying, naturally, to move out even more of the stool left in the rest of his bowel.

He began suffering abdominal cramps.

By the time his plane landed, the cramping was painful enough for his wife to take him to the hospital. The doctors took a report from him, asking what had happened to him in the last twenty-four hours. He told them he had received colon hydrotherapy.

They diagnosed his problem as a perforated bowel, resulting from the colon cleansing.

In a panic, the cancer-sufferer's wife called the doctor in San Diego who had referred the patient to me. She hysterically explained what had transpired. Coincidentally, I was working in the referring doctor's office, so I answered the phone and caught the brunt of the poor woman's frustration, fear, and anger.

Even as I sympathized, all I could imagine was a huge lawsuit. I knew I had done nothing harmful, but with the medical prejudices against internal cleansing, I did not believe I would have a chance. I could not understand it; when he left my office, this sick man had been feeling so much better!

The M.D. who had referred the patient to me called the hospital, identified himself with his medical credentials, and asked to speak to the diagnosing doctors. He explained that he had prescribed the colon hydrotherapy. After talking with this M.D., the hospital's doctors CHANGED THEIR DIAGNOSIS. The man was given treatment for his exaggerated symptoms, and all turned out well.

This incident was not caused by the hospital doctors' ignorance. They knew the cancer victim did not have a perforated colon. But because of prejudice, they decided to blame colon hydrotherapy.

The diagnosis was retracted only when it was found out a fellow M.D. had prescribed treatment. Otherwise, the previous diagnosis would have stuck. No one would have known any different. The establishment could have said anything it wanted, and no one could have questioned it.

The reader should note that after administering approximately twenty-five thousand treatments of internal cleansing, not ONE of my clients has ever experienced a perforated colon or any other problems resulting from internal cleansing!

Paralysis gone

Dear Millan:
I came to you because I had arthritis in my right hip. I felt like I weighed 600 lbs. and dragged around with a cane until it felt as if I was wearing out my shoulders from leaning on the cane. In June and July 1994, I got shots of cortisone in the right hip that caused more pain. In October, I went to another Rheumatologist that gave me Indocin. A few days later, I was so sick I thought I would die and went to urgent care. I waited such a long time. When the doctor finally came in, he said I had a virus.

Then I decided to get colonics. After seven colonics, I began to see movement in the right side of my face, which had been paralyzed for 20 years because of a brain tumor.

I had no idea that it could improve. After the eighth colonic, we went out to get a sandwich and I finished before my husband did. This was a surprise because for 20 years I was uncomfortable at dinner parties because I was always the last one to finish, when everyone else's plates were cleared away. This was because of the paralysis on my face. My right hip has improved a lot and I go without the cane; still limited but soooo much better. I am off all the pills for arthritis and all laxatives.

Thank you so much,
Helen

Positive comments by Medical Doctors

In his work, a Dr. Kennedy states: putrefying waste material causes autointoxication and leads to dangerous pre-cancerous conditions in the colon. In addition, various other gastrointestinal complaints and diseases are associated with a poisoned bowel.

Dr. John W. Travis, MD stated: I believe colon therapy is one of many important forms of treatment that we were not taught in medical school.

Bessie Jo Tillman, M.D., of Redding, also wrote:

I frequently refer [constipated] patients for colon [hydro] therapy... I have never had problems with serious injuries and illnesses, such as infection, bowel perforation, bowel necrosis (death of the bowel tissues caused by use of caustic soaps or other irritants that attack the delicate lining of the colon) and death with the sophisticated and refined temperatures and pressure gauges, disposable tubing and speculum and trained certified therapists... I have only obtained positive results. I have never had complaints.

Elson M. Haas, M.D., director of a clinic in San Rafael, states that in over fifteen years of referring patients to colon hydrotherapists for treatment, he has "never seen any medical complications... in over hundreds of patients."

He goes on to explain the safety and efficacy of modern internal cleansing practices, and ultimately maintains, "There is essentially no risk of medical problems."

And again, "[This] simple procedure cannot cause bowel necrosis and death, and in well-trained hands with proper techniques there is no risk of infection and bowel perforation."

Paul Lynn, M.D., of San Francisco, had this to say: "I have frequently referred patients to get [internal cleansing] from a qualified therapist [who] uses proven sophisticated equipment including a refined pressure gauge along with disposable tubing. I have received only positive reports from these sessions and if it were not safe and sanitary, I would not recommend them."

Invasive procedure?
Doctors have objected to internal cleansing as an invasive procedure; however, is not brushing our

teeth an invasive procedure, getting a tattoo, douching, putting a Q-tip in your ears, or inserting a suppository?

Medical doctors oftentimes cannot guarantee positive results from their invasive procedures. On the other hand, qualified colon hydrotherapists can be sure what their clients receive is not "an element of the practice of medicine which has been outlawed."

Take Charge of Personal Health

Unless more physicians and their patients are educated about internal cleansing and its real health benefits, it is likely someone in the medical establishment will again try to rob the populace of this legitimate health option.

Knowledge is victory over victimization and illness. Individuals must seek out their own best health! They must take control over their own bodies.

People can begin today to live in optimum health through colon cleansing, cleansing herbs, and proper diet.

Approximately, ten thousand people a week get colonics in the United States.

CHAPTER SIX

Quote: To be a good leader, you must be able to serve your fellow man.
Millan Chessman

AILMENTS OF THE DIGESTIVE SYSTEM AND CAUSES

Can you find your pet ailment, complaint, or medical condition among the following health problems?

Bad breath (despite proper oral hygiene), chronic skin dryness or blemishes, sallow skin, lifeless, dull hair (not due to chemical over-processing, such as bleaching, coloring or perming), psoriasis, and nail fungus.

Testimonial

My testimonial: Millan Chessman

After 35 years of having fungus on my toe nail and after trying everything to no avail, I started dipping "food grade hydrogen peroxide" on my toenail and in 3 months a new nail started growing and now I have no more fungus.

Nail fungus, for example, is nearly impossible to heal. Patients serious about eradicating it completely, rather than spending money on endless preparations that do not work and the time and inevitable pain as the nail is eaten away, often submit to podiatrists who usually have no choice but to suggest removal of the nails.

But before taking that radical step, one patient, Richard, went the following route of internal cleansing:

Testimonial

Fungus

I went to the podiatrist because I had fungus on my toenails. He initially told me it would take eight months for this fungus to clear up, and he only gave a sixty percent success rate if I had the toenails removed.

He wanted to give me a prescription, stating the drug did have side effects and it was very expensive, $2.50 a pill.

I refused and went the internal cleansing route. Shortly after, I started internal cleansing. I also changed my diet and took lactobacillus acidophilus and received lactobacillus acidophilus-bifidus implants at the end of my colon cleansing sessions.

'I then went back to the doctor. He was amazed and stated that the progress I made in this month was remarkable.

Signed,
Richard

The Symptoms Keep Coming

If a person has or has had one or more of the following health problems, perhaps the state of the health of the colon should be seriously considered.

Practically all chronic, and most acute, physical and physiological ailments can be at least partially traced back to an unhealthy bowel. All these ailments can be adversely affected by a sick, clogged colon.

These problems could be gall bladder problems, liver problems not due to cirrhosis or hepatitis, tendencies toward nicotine, drug, alcohol, or caffeine addictions, basic immune deficiency (not the genetic condition or AIDS), chronic susceptibility to illness, and hormonal imbalances. Indigestion, "nervous bowel," or irritable bowel syn-

72

drome, constipation, diarrhea, hemorrhoids, Diverticulosis, or diverticulitis, frequent use of laxatives or products such as Kaopectate or Pepto-Bismol, and offensive, persistent body odor, despite daily bathing and hygiene.

There is more; get the picture?

Testimonial

Epilepsy Disappears

Dear Millan:

I want to thank you and Judy for being your competent, professional and caring selves. Your treatments were very effective, and we believe I have now become completely cured of my epilepsy condition that has plagued me over the past year. My system feels much different and I feel healthier than I have in a long time. Your program was vital for complete success. Thank you and Judy for being there. Here's wishing you the very best in life,

Love,
Dave G.

Back Pain and Other Common Ailments

Joint pain, gout, high blood pressure, atherosclerosis, and high cholesterol; my clients who have suffered from chronic sciatica, pain or numbness in lower extremities, or unexplained back pain, have stated they have experienced relief through internal cleansing.

Chronic back pain of mysterious origin plagues countless, otherwise healthy, people, often resulting in disability so severe they cannot do the simplest things or hold down jobs.

Even with diagnosable causes, doctors can do little, short of experimental surgery, to ease the pain. Many back surgeries are unsuccessful in achieving that aim.

Certainly, a heavily impacted and poisonous colon contributes to the problem, as it puts pressure on the sciatic and lumbar nerves. But this aspect is almost universally overlooked by conventional physicians.

One of the symptoms of worms and parasites is a backache.

Chiropractors can make adjustments that can help. But, more important, internal cleansing, with the detoxification program, has helped many clients. The following is a letter from one such client:

Testimonial

Back Pain Disappeared

I have a fifth lumbar vertebra, which is cracked on one side and crushed on the other. For ten years, I suffered mornings upon arising because of pressure on the fifth vertebra. When getting out of bed, I would have to walk for ten to fifteen minutes until the discomfort would go away.

I cannot explain it, but after doing internal cleansing sessions and the cleansing program, this pain in the back disappeared and I have not had it since.

Signed,
Winnie

Addiction

It makes sense that an inefficient digestive system would encourage addictions. When the colon is clogged with rotting garbage, it cannot get rid of toxins. In fact, these poisons are reabsorbed into the body. In turn, the body, under attack by poisons and out of balance, seeks ways of hastening absorption, and the brain seeks chemical relief.

Clients stated that internal cleansing and detoxification have alleviated their toxic conditions by enabling the body to kick addictive habits.

Addiction is a process of habituation over a period of weeks, months, or, more often, years.

Withdrawal is difficult and usually painful, both psychologically and physically. Rehabilitation programs often do not work because this transition to non-addiction is so painful, including violent fevers, sweating, and weakness with muscular contractions and uncontrollable trembling, nausea, and diarrhea.

These excruciating and humiliating symptoms last anywhere from a few hours to a few days, and the residual psychological craving can hang on for torturous years. Counseling and support groups are nice, but are too often inadequate for the addict's ultimate success.

Internal cleansing, with a detoxification program, should be considered as a definite means to break the addiction.

During the body's natural cleansing process, all foreign matter is sent to the liver for detoxification. From there it is delivered to the excretory organs, the kidneys and the digestive tract via bile, for elimination from the body.

A slow-moving, unhealthy colon causes reabsorption of the drug-laden bile. To break the reabsorption cycle, the waste products stored in the large bowel must be evacuated.

A detoxification cleansing program and internal cleansing performs just this function, with the added benefit that it stimulates a sluggish colon to begin normal peristalsis. Internal cleansing can assist in an efficient, gentle way to help the addict with his addiction. I believe internal cleansing should be a required step in any drug rehabilitation program.

Even years later, the effects of drug use can be purged from the body. One client commented that she had smoked pot regularly for a short period in her youth, but that she had not partaken for ten years.

She went through a cleansing program of a juice fast, internal cleansing sessions and herbal cleansers. On this regimen, she experienced a mild high, as if she were stoned on pot.

It could be that the THC, or tetrahydrocan-nabinol, was stored in her fat cells and other tissues for many years, and started releasing into the bloodstream and being eliminated out of her body. Why else would she feel high?

Another client who had been a heroin addict said she had not used heroin for fifteen years. When she did a cleansing program with internal cleansing, she said she could actually smell the unique odor of the heroin seep out of the pores of her skin.

Medical studies have shown that certain insoluble chemicals can indeed be stored in fat cells and other tissues, sometimes to deadly effect, as with DDT.

Testimonial

Nasal Spray Addiction Gone

Even over-the-counter drugs can build up toxins in the body and may lead to dependence on the substance. Here is the case of one man's experience with nasal spray:

I was taking nasal spray for twenty-four years. I was doing up to one twelve-hour bottle a week, spraying every two hours. I could never get off it without having severe side effects, such as nasal swelling, fever, throat swelling, and basic inability to breathe.

While doing the colon cleansing program and after my second internal cleansing session, I went off the spray. I have had absolutely no problems and have been off it ever since.

Signed, Robert

Another client, a former alcoholic who was sober for twelve years, had a series of internal cleansing sessions coupled with the dietary and herbal cleansing programs. Soon after, his body began to reek of stale booze. The odor eventually went away as all the garbage was finally eliminated from his body. The process was quite an experience!

The Dotolo Institute states the following:

Recent observations proved that internal cleansing is very beneficial as part of a drug rehabilitation program, insofar as test persons indicated a considerable reduction in the craving for addictive drugs. A closely controlled test series in drug-rehabilitation centers is being prepared at present.

Internal cleansing and Substance Rehabilitation

Drugs decrease bowel activity and cocaine and its myriad derivatives are absorbed at a much higher rate than the liver can filter out.

So many clients that I have seen over the years have stated that they have gotten rid of their addictions doing a cleansing program.

Testimonial

Overcame Drug and Alcohol Abuse

I have a tremendous background of drug abuse. You name it, and I did it. I also drank very heavily. I am now forty years old, and I felt detoxification and internal cleansing would help me. I read about it and did a series with Millan.

With her supervision in my juice fasting, colon hydrotherapy, and taking the cleansing herbs, I was shocked to see all this sewage come out of my body. I think what really shocked me was even after my seventh session; the smell of the stool which came out of my body was wretched. It was unbelievable after that many treatments!

Signed, Will

Diabetes

Several experiences with diabetics seem to point to internal cleansing programs as a way to lessen the effects of the disease. Diabetics have claimed victory over the devastating consequences of this often progressively debilitating disease, which can lead to blindness, kidney failure, gangrene with amputation of feet and legs, and, of course, premature death.

If the true aim of medicine is to alleviate as much undue suffering as possible when an absolute cure may not be attainable, then the response of diabetic conditions to internal cleansing should be looked at closely by the medical community.

Testimonial

Diabetes Blood Sugar Level Normalized

This story from Charles highlights the point:

Before internal cleansing, I was diagnosed with Type II diabetes. My blood sugar level averaged 150 to 180 every morning. Sometimes it went as high as 300 when I ate donuts. But I found out that these levels were dangerous.

I started internal cleansing, with the internal cleansing program. After the sixth colon cleansing session, my blood sugar level dropped to an average of 100 and then became normal, even though during my series I blew it twice by eating donuts! I tested my blood level when I did this and it had not gone up!

I tried to believe that I was cured of diabetes, but I know I was not. I know I must watch my diet.

Doctors tell diabetics to watch their diets, but that is easier said than done. It is like telling a drug addict not to do drugs. I know how much the internal cleansing helped keep my cravings for sugar down.

Internal cleansing has made all the difference in my eating habits, especially my cravings. Overall, my energy has increased and I feel great.

Signed,
Charles

It is perfectly logical that what goes into your body must affect it; otherwise, we would not need to eat, period. Because this is not a perfect world, we live in intimate contact with harmful microorganisms and potentially toxic chemicals - many of which are made and given off even by otherwise benign microorganisms. This happens in our own digestive system.

Testimonial

Diabetic's Story

I had diabetes for seventeen years. My kidneys were not functioning correctly. Protein leaked into my urine instead of needy areas of my body. As a result, my tissues swelled with fluid. I gained twenty pounds. I swelled up so dangerously I was admitted to the hospital. There, the doctors had me taking sixteen of the strongest type of water pills a day.

While taking these pills, I saw spots, white dots, became dizzy and had a fast heartbeat. My doctor told me in five years I would be dead from kidney failure. I felt so bad I believed him. He asked if I had problems seeing. If so, he said, my eyes had developed lesions. When your kidneys go, your eyesight also goes. I got worse because I was frightened, and I believed what he was saying. Then I got angry. I said to him, "Only God will determine my death, not you, doctor!"

Over a period of a few months, my determination to beat this thing changed. I prayed a lot, changed my eating habits, started exercising, moved to a new home, and started an internal cleansing program.

I was going through a detoxification stage. I developed cold-like symptoms.

My BUN (a test of kidney function) was seventy-five when I was ill and in the hospital. After the cleansing program, it went down to nineteen. The optimum level is seventeen.

I remember my doctor had told me I would never improve, and it was a matter of time for my kidneys to totally fail! If he could only see me now!

Signed,
Sally

Cholesterol

Dr. William Welles, author of *The Shocking Truth about Cholesterol,* also asserts that the bile routes must remain unclogged because bile regulates cholesterol:

Cholesterol levels can actually be regulated by the body itself through the liver, provided that bile has a chance to act on fat. When bile breaks down fat the liver can then convert excess cholesterol into bile for future use.

When you ingest fat, the gall bladder contracts, releasing bile for digestion.

Testimonial

Help with High Cholesterol

Dear Millan:
I started your cleansing program and my cholesterol went from 286 down to 204. I lost 18 pounds and the cleansing gave me control of eating the wrong foods. I got away from eating animals, sugar and white flour.
The doctor did a blood test after – lipid panels, everything went down to normal. I didn't want to take prescription drugs before deciding to do the internal cleansing. Now I eat natural foods. The doctor asked me "What are you doing because you look great?" I told him I am doing colonic hydrotherapy.

Sincerely,
Darlene

According to Welles, the bile is then reabsorbed further down the digestive tract.

If the colon is constipated, still more bile re-absorption takes place. The liver is signaled to produce less bile, with the consequence that less cholesterol is converted to

80

bile and more is dangerously released into the bloodstream.

This indicates that often high cholesterol is less related to how much fat you eat but more to how well your colon is working; in other words, how much bile your liver can produce by cholesterol conversion.

The importance of a well-functioning, properly moving colon cannot be overemphasized. You ignore it or mistreat it at your peril.

There are six channels of elimination in the body: skin, colon, lymph, kidneys, lungs and liver.

Testimonial

Kidney Problem Resolved

Julie's kidneys hurt so that she could barely walk or touch her back. Her urine stung, and she had to push it out. After the second session, all pain went away. Amazingly, her back felt better.

She exercised more, drank more water, and was eating healthier. She had gone two weeks without bowel movements, and she had headaches every day. After a number of sessions, she had bowel movements regularly and no headaches. After the tenth session, she passed two white strands, one long and white, and the other shorter, which a lab later determined to be worms. She was very sick, but afterwards she received another session, which relieved her discomfort.

Signed,
Julie

Colon Cancer

Most colon therapists are convinced, as I certainly am, that the great increase in colon cancer over the past few generations is also due to autointoxication in the colon. High fiber foods change the bacterial flora of your colon to non-carcinogenic organisms and drastically reduce the possibility of colon cancer.

Medical doctors are simply not trained to deal with the colon until it becomes severely diseased. I tell my clients the prevention of disease begins with an internal cleansing program. This is invaluable.

A client told me she went to the doctor and asked about some mucus she saw in her bowel movement. She wondered why he replied that the discharge came not from her bowel but from her vagina. I, too, wondered why the doctor did not seem to know mucus is found numerous times in stool.

Testimonial

Prostate Cancer Recovery

Dear Millan,

I was diagnosed with prostate cancer, and I decided to go the wholistic route instead of orthodox medicine. My wife prepared me organic vegetable and fruit juices, which I drank exclusively a total of thirty days.

I took cleansing herbs and did colon hydrotherapy every other day.

After thirty days, I went back to my doctor and the tests were negative. There was no sign of cancer. I am the happiest man in the world.

Signed,
Raymond

Which treatment would you rather have...internal cleansing, chemotherapy, radiation, or surgery?

Which is more unnatural?

Which one has more unnatural effects?

Which one restores a more natural state of health?

What if everyone tried internal cleansing first? What might happen?

One of my clients takes a very balanced, pragmatic view. While conceding that internal cleansing may not be natural in that birds and beasts do not practice it, he also acknowledges that internal cleansing is necessary in our society today. He knows it is difficult, nearly impossible, to avoid most harmful chemicals, preservatives, and pesticides, even with his efforts at determinedly maintaining a good diet. He points out that as long as there are unnatural, unhealthful additives in the environment, he will combat them with a harmless but effective colon cleanse, however "unnatural" it seems.

This client comes regularly to have his body cleansed and refreshed on the inside.

He has taken proactive steps to maintaining his own health - his life.

Testimonial

Cancer Survivor

I had a malignant tumor on my lymph node. The medical doctor wanted to remove it surgically, and proceed with chemo and radiation. I chose the alternative route.

I started internal cleansing with Millan Chessman. She put me on an herbal cleansing program and colonics once a week. My diet consisted of vegetables, fruits, grains, legumes, raw nuts and seeds. I did skin brushing two times a day.

After having the cleansing sessions with Millan, my malignant tumor is completely gone. I couldn't help but get emotional with tears at the discovery.

Signed,
Michael K.

Colon cancer is the first leading cause of cancer deaths in the United States. Every fifty-six seconds, an American is being diagnosed with cancer in the United States.

If we as a society adopted internal cleansing as a second-line (the first being proper diet), disease prevention strategy, many such deaths could be avoided.

Colorectal Cancer

Finally, the most dreaded and devastating of possible colon ailments: colorectal cancer.

In the alimentary canal, the most common cancers are stomach cancer and colorectal cancer. The latter disease is almost exclusively a phenomenon of the Western world, with the highest incidence reported in the United States. It is now recognized that colorectal cancer is directly linked to a high animal low-fiber diet.

Colorectal cancer is found in the area at the beginning of the colon, or at the site of the sigmoid and rectum; hence, the compound name of the disease, colorectal.

This fatal disease claims the lives of over sixty thousand people annually.

Testimonial

Lump on Breast Completely Gone

Dear Millan,
I had a lump about one inch in diameter on my breast. It was painful, and I became very concerned.

I then went on the fasting program, taking cleansing herbs, and doing colon hydrotherapy each day.

I am excited to tell you the lump is completely gone. Why aren't more people doing this wonderful program? I have never felt better in my life.
Signed,
Millie

Respiratory Disease

The process of digestion requires the cooperation of microorganisms living in our bowels, and with-

84

out which we cannot live. We depend on these tiny creatures to digest our food and release its nutrients into our bloodstream.

The aorta, the large artery leading directly from the heart, picks up nutrients from the intestine and distributes them to all parts of the body. Since one of its vital distribution points is the lungs, respiratory disease should be linked to digestion more often than not.

Chronic bronchitis, a common ailment of the respiratory system, is a response to environmental and internal toxins. When medical treatments, focusing on symptoms, cannot clear it up, it is logical to look for causes from within the body itself. The supply post for toxins is the colon.

Fermenting, decaying waste material is sent out into the bloodstream by the out-of-control E. coli II, which have taken over the clogged colon. Wide-ranging results follow, as the case of Frank clearly shows:

Testimonial

Energy & Stamina Increased

In the spring, I developed bronchitis. By November, I was at my wit's end because nothing I did made it any better.

When I read that an impacted colon blocks the normal elimination systems of the body, causing a backup of toxins to the organs, I questioned if it applied to my situation. The article highlighted the mucus deposits in the lungs as a breeding ground for bacteria and resulting respiratory problems.

I decided to try a colon-cleansing series. Within two days, the bronchitis disappeared.

The health benefits I have gained from bi-annual internal cleansing treatments have been beyond my greatest expectations. As my organs regained their health, the puffiness, lines, and other indications of advancing age lessened. My energy

85

and stamina increased each year. My mental awareness and creativity are noticeably stronger after a series of internal cleansings.

Signed,
Frank

Internal cleansing has also been a source of emotional release. Every emotional experience causes a chemical response in the body. Those chemicals are stored in the tissues when they cannot be effectively eliminated and are toxic to those tissues. Besides storing toxins, the tissues are typically deficient in necessary minerals because the walls of an impacted colon are unable to absorb them.

The bottom line of internal cleansing is that it eliminates all the accumulated toxins and allows proper absorption and distribution of the vital minerals to all the tissues. Another important benefit of internal cleansing is hydration, as most people are dehydrated. Some feel that is the number one benefit.

My Daughter's Recovery from Allergies

My daughter Roxanne had terrible allergies and was taking those horrible shots to combat it. The MD said it was the worst case of allergies he had seen in 25 years of practice. I kept telling her, "Honey, just clean out your body and change your diet and your allergies will go away."

She would say, "Oh, mother, it is not my colon, it is the pollen and cat hair I am allergic to." So one night she came home (her husband and she were living with me at the time) and said she was going to go on a spiritual fast for five days because she had just become a born-again Christian and wanted to draw closer to Jesus. I immediately started giving her cleansing herbs and the second day she did internal colon cleansing. She was shocked to see what came out of her body. She continued with more colon cleansing sessions. She never had the allergies again. Today, she herself

86

is a very successful colon hydrotherapist. You know our children, they never believe their mothers! She commented on how lovely her skin looked, because before she had blemishes around her chin area.

Testimonial

Acne Gone

For you sufferers of that scourge of young skin, let us discuss acne. A young lady in her mid-twenties came to me for internal cleansing. Her intent was to get rid of a bad case of pimples.

Her boyfriend had heard about internal cleansing and suggested she try it.

She did a series of ten internal cleansing sessions. By her sixth session, she started to see her skin clear up. When she came in for her seventh session, she was ecstatic. She looked lovely, and her boyfriend was so happy with at how nice she looked.

By the time she completed her series, her skin was totally cleared up. Her unnecessary misery had been contributed to by a simple cause: a malfunctioning colon, which began to poison her body and betrayed itself in her skin. She also had a history of previous drug abuse.

Anonymous

Parasites and Worms

Parasites and worms are another largely overlooked health threat in the United States. Dr. Zane Gard, M.D., and other doctors estimate that approximately ninety percent of our population unknowingly harbors worms and parasites of one sort or another.

Worms are given the opportunity to invade the body through bad hygiene. Amoebas may ulcerate the walls of the colon and invade the circulatory system, where they are distributed everywhere in the body.

People can contract parasites and worms through water, air, and foods such as meats, fish, chicken, fruits, vegetables, even organic vegetables, pets and other people.

A nurse told me an elderly man came to their office because he was having problems in his ear and wanted it checked. After checking his ear, the doctor fell against the wall in total shock. Inside the ear was a maggot!

Another client told me she purchased fish, fresh from the fish market, came home and proceeded to prepare it. Lo and behold worms, many of them coming through the flesh of the fish. She then took it back to the fish market and complained and the butcher told her "oh that is so common, we see this all of the time. We just simply scrape the worms off. Don't worry, when you cook it, it will kill all of the worms". I don't think so...not me!

Another client told me after she had her sixth colonic, she went home feeling very bloated and uncomfortable. That evening she went to the bathroom and mucus came out of her with a number of worms in it. After passing that she felt much better and the bloating subsided.

Getting water to the beginning of the colon at the cecum is very important because that critical spot is where the worms and parasites reside. One 28 year old woman was sent to me by her M.D. for a series of cleanses after he diagnosed that she had an infestation of two types of amoeba parasites. She can attest to the importance of this type of treatment.

The woman came in for a series of cleansing sessions. She later passed a beef tapeworm and the M.D. did not even know that she had it in her body. She continued with cleansing sessions.

Another woman came to me after she coughed up what she thought was mucus, but turned out to be a live worm squirming out of her mouth.

Another client came to me after she had an infestation, when after a session, she accidentally passed a worm-filled puddle on the bathroom floor. They were alive and wiggling.

Some health authorities estimate the majority of our population harbors worms and other parasites, which remain undetected.

Symptoms are identical to myriads of other ailments. It is important to not establish a positive diagnosis without complete testing by professionals.

Moreover, infestation will aggravate other existing maladies. We offer special tests to detect infestations. These involve examination of stool coming out from the ninth purge, and there are other clinics specializing in this as well.

Testimonial

Tapeworm Discovered

Dear Millan:

Diagnosed as having two different types of amoebas, I came to you for help. After the thirteenth treatment, I passed a flat noodle-like substance. Laboratory analysis revealed it a beef tapeworm. My doctor had performed numerous tests on me, yet had not discovered this creature. Thank you for your help.

Anonymous

It is not the norm for us to go to the medical doctor and have stool examined for worms or parasites. Yet this is a very common problem and we do not want to face its possibility. We do not hesitate to consent to the vet's checking our animals (pets) for this condition, yet our diet is as bad as theirs. Heaven forbid we have worms or parasites!

89

I remember an incident many years ago before I knew much about good health, which occurred during a two week trip with my family. One hour before we left, my son unplugged the freezer to plug in the iron, and forgot to plug the freezer back in. The freezer was full of meat of all kinds located in a tightly sealed storage room. When we got home after entering the attached garage, the odor hit us! What is that smell??? It was horrible! The big shock came after we opened to door to the storage room. This little room was full of flies. How did they get in when everything was closed up tight as a drum? The freezer was loaded with maggots. But from where? This meat had to have the eggs in there to begin with.

Another time, my mother took some red snapper fish out of the freezer, and marinated it as it defrosted on the counter. This was going to be our dinner that evening. The fish, however, was full of worms wiggling all over, after it defrosted. Just recently I watched a program on people with worms and the "parasitologist" stated "freezing your fish will kill the worms." That is simply not true!

We think nothing of eating raw fish in the form of sushi. Do we have any idea what we are putting into our bodies? Yes there possibly are parasites, and or eggs, in our vegetables, but you can eliminate that problem that immersing the veggies and fruits in hydrogen peroxide for 40 minutes. Put 2 tablespoons into 1 gallon of water. This will lift larvae, pesticides, chemicals, etc.

Numerous times, while administering colonics, I have seen tiny worms wiggling in the anal area of my client. Itching in the anal area could be a sign of worms. It was discovered in an autopsy that a lady who had complained of severe headaches actually housed larvae in her brain. An optometrist told me that once in an eye examination he saw a worm dash from the patient's pupil, going back behind the eyeball.

So often a normal stool sample will not reveal worms or parasites. It would have to be a severe case in order for this condition to be diagnosed. That is because the cecum is where worms nest which is at the beginning of the colon, near the appendix.

Constipation

The colon itself can suffer acute or chronic conditions. Probably the most familiar to all of us is constipation. This is often the first telltale sign of bad eating habits; however, the cause is blatantly overlooked because our American culture takes for granted harmful dietary intake.

In short, constipation, derived from a Latin word meaning to press, crowd together, pack, or cram, is exactly that - a colon packed with old drying fecal matter it has not been allowed to, or cannot, evacuate.

Constipation is caused directly by the following: an unhealthy diet consisting of too much animal, dairy products, cooked and processed foods, bad elimination habits and posture, drinking too little water, high stress levels, especially for women, illegal drugs and legal, over-the-counter or prescription drugs, laxatives, lack of proper balance of vital intestinal bacteria, lack of exercise, cultural stigma in certain situations, and weakness of the abdominal muscles that aid evacuation. Other causes are low thyroid, gall bladder problems, and a dysfunctional liver.

Constipation can be a leading cause of disease and disease susceptibility. As previously stated, the longer rotting waste material stays in the body, the more toxins are produced. More tissues are broken down by toxic action, which either store or excrete the toxins.

The body's defenses weaken as its arsenal is concentrated on internal adversaries rather than elements invading from the outside. Constipation reduces the body to this state, acting as an open invitation for disease - including colorectal cancer.

91

I tell my clients that if they think they are not constipated because they may have one or two bowel movements a day, "Think again!" I tell them, "If your diet is unhealthy, no matter how often you defecate, you may still have an impacted colon. Your colon may have waste matter trapped in excess mucus - produced by your desperate intestine which tries to trap and therefore neutralize all the bad stuff."

Testimonial

Bloating & Constipation

I recently went through an internal cleansing program, and my health improved! I was tired, my stomach ached and was bloated, and constipation was a problem.
My doctor recommended internal cleansing, so I did not waste any time getting started. The colon hydrotherapist guided me through the program. The more she explained to me, the more it made sense
I feel as if for years I have been mistreating my body. Now that I understand, I know many people out there suffer needlessly. I feel great.

Anonymous

Hemorrhoids

Before we move on, one more direct result of constipation must be addressed. This is hemorrhoids. Hemorrhoids, or piles, are not caused by reading on the toilet. Hemorrhoids are caused by straining at the toilet to eliminate during constipation. It is common to see them in internal cleansing.

The pressure, both from the obvious weight and bulk of the accumulated feces and from muscles striving to push the hardened matter out, also pushes out, literally inverting, the inner lining and tissues of the anal sphincters.

The constriction is so severe on the delicate tissues and their capillaries that it ruptures many of them, causing localized internal - and sometimes external - bleeding, an obvious invitation for infection. It produces what are essentially varicose veins in the anus.

"Piles" are the pockets of blood and damaged tissues that make up hemorrhoids. They often protrude outside the anus when having a bowel movement. As you may know, this condition is extremely painful. The huge amounts of Preparation H and such remedies and the brisk sales of "tush cushions" testify to its prevalence.

My clients have stated this condition was improved by simply taking proper care of their colon through diet and cleansing.

Thanks to our cultural attitude toward the bowels, it is little known or acknowledged that straining at the toilet is also a leading cause of sudden death and fatal heart attack, especially among the elderly. Many collapse and die right on the toilet.

The Urge to Defecate

How many of us have been out in a restaurant, airport, or any public place and have had the urge to defecate?

But the average person says, "No, I cannot go now." This person chooses to wait until getting home where it is more private. Elimination is just more comfortable in one's own home, rather than a public place.

It is important that when people feel the urge to have a bowel movement, they go immediately. If they do not go, then their lack of response will cause their colon not to prompt them as frequently as it has in the past.

Again, it is our culture that places us in this situation. We feel ashamed and embarrassed that someone will hear us, and we do not want to offend because of the foul odor the waste produces.

This retention contributes to constipation. Then, when we do go to the bathroom, we strain.

Since the stool is very hard, we have two problems: constipation and hemorrhoids.

One out of every two people I see has a hemorrhoid. It is a very common condition. The quicker people learn to eliminate, the better and healthier they will be.

Also, people must be sure that when they do go to the bathroom they are not rushed. One needs to stay on the toilet until completely finished.

With some people, fifteen minutes should be allowed on the toilet. If it is difficult to go, one can take a good book, something positive like a Bible, and read it on the toilet. Before long, a person will be going regularly.

A person should go even if no urge is felt. It will happen. Sitting on the toilet at the same time daily will encourage the body to respond. We are creatures of habit. So the idea that haste makes waste in this case does not apply.

Waste products become impacted in the pockets of the colon, especially in the diverticula (those little pouches that hang like baggy growths on the walls of the colon). As more and more fecal matter becomes trapped, the center tunnel, where a limited amount of waste is allowed to pass, becomes more and more distorted, resulting in restrictive passage flow, even though elimination may occur twice a day.

In his book, *Become Younger*, Dr. Walker tells how in an autopsy he saw a colon, which measured eleven inches in diameter, with a central passageway in the encrusted fecal matter of only the diameter of a pencil.

There is another danger in the mucoid fecal matter that builds up in an unhealthy colon: it provides a perfect breeding ground for harmful bacteria, and is a reservoir for all the harmful toxins the bacteria produce. Importantly, it is a pathway of disease agents resulting from poisons and free radicals. Opsudo memberiouses is a false membrane, formed as a response to too many antibiotics, which interferes with normal bowel flora and function.

Gary N. Lewkovich, D.C., cites eight reasons individuals develop constipation:

1. *Too little fiber in the diet.*
   (Animal Products have NO fiber).
2. *Too little water consumed.*
3. *Too little exercise.*
4. *Too much stress.*
5. *Poor elimination habits.*
6. *Certain prescription drugs.*
7. *Certain foods.*
8. *Certain pathologies affecting the lower digestive tract.*

You cannot afford a clogged colon. Constipation is a serious condition that demands immediate attention if you desire good health. Your colon hydrotherapist can provide the path to good health.

This leads to clogged conditions in other vital digestive systems as well.

Rich Anderson, author of *Cleanse and Purify Thyself*, went through a number of fasts and colon cleansings. He became amazed with the long strands of ropy mucoidal matter he saw coming out of him in the view-tube during internal cleansing.

Anderson attempted to categorize the consistent shapes and sizes of the mucoid fecal matter, based on the theory that the shapes of the pieces would indicate their origin in the intestine, in the same way that Play-Doh conforms to impressions. He thought that he could identify the sections of colon to which the slimy goo had been molded. The duration of colon impaction might be determined by the distance into the intestine. He states:

> *If your colon has been impacted for some time, the body's natural defense against all the junk is to produce mucus to try to help trap it and move it out.*

The small intestine may become involved in producing this excess mucus. When that happens, the bile ducts may become blocked. Anderson states that if that happens, the essential bile fluids produced by the liver will not be able to reach the food for proper digestion and assimilation.

Bacterial and chemical chaos will ensue, with dire results as outlined in the previous discussion. Thus, the stage is set for all kinds of malfunctions and diseases, including precancerous and cancerous.

Testimonial

Severe Constipation Gone

Dear Millan:

I want to thank you for everything you have done for me. You really have changed my life.

Before I met you I was your average processed food eating, unhealthy, overweight, constipated person. I really cannot remember being regular. After not having a bowel movement for one month, unsuccessful laxative prescriptions and a painful barium enema test, I was told there was nothing wrong with me and I still had not gone to the bathroom! It was then that colonics was recommended to me. I was very hesitant at first but was at a point where I would try anything because I had experienced so much discomfort. Now after nine colonics, with one more to go, I can absolutely say I am more healthy, happy and energized than ever before.

I have lost over 10 pounds, have absolutely no craving for sugar or carbohydrates, and feel like weight has been lifted off my entire body. I can honestly say that I never thought I could feel so refreshed. I feel like many toxins have been removed from my system and feel younger than I have in a long time.

Along with your highly recommended

change in diet, I think this cleansing program has benefited me more over the past 10 weeks than any other weight loss program or system ever could. I know now I can be healthy for the rest of my life. I still have more weight to lose, but with your advice and coaching, I know I can be as fit as I want to be. I have a family history of colon cancer and obesity. I have learned now that I can overcome these diseases and live a long and healthy life.

I have received so many compliments over the past few weeks it is amazing! I hope you know that you really have changed my life and I FEEL I HAVE NO WAY OF THANKING YOU ENOUGH. I definitely plan to maintain a fitness and health program including colonics and I hope you will be available to help me out in the future. Thank you very Much.

Signed, Michele D.F.

Laxatives

Frequent use of laxatives, even the "bulking" ones, actually contributes to constipation, the very condition it purports to eliminate.

Most laxatives work by chemically poisoning and irritating the lining of the colon, the very tissue and muscle that channels nutrients and wastes from the bloodstream. Naturally, the irritated colon heaves in super-agitated contractions in a desperate attempt to get rid of the offending laxatives. Anything loose enough to flow out with the resulting diarrhea will be expelled.

This emergency rush of watery stool is really massive dehydration. Dehydration of the colon produces constipation. So, the vicious cycle continues, with the consequent need for possibly another stronger laxative dose.

Several things happen: the chronically constipated colon comes to depend on the irritant stimulus of the laxative to contract for defecation. This causes a dependence on the laxative, the laxative causes dehydration, dehydration causes constipation, and dependence on laxatives causes the colon to become ever more weakened. Even herbal laxatives can cause the colon to become dependent on them.

A standard American diet, combined with various medications, causes an aging bowel to get tired and just give up. Chronic sufferers of constipation were always middle-aged or elderly, but now the young suffer as well.

The real beneficiaries of laxatives are those who make and sell them. The financial success of these companies and their distributors is clear evidence that we Westerners are having a collective colon crisis; therefore, it is clear that internal cleansing, which contributes to good health, is vitally needed and should be implemented.

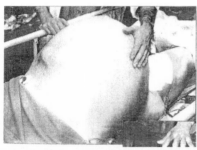
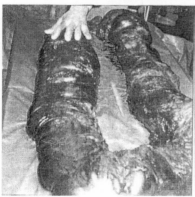

Diarrhea refers to bowel movements that occur too often and are too loose. Diarrhea can be caused by impacted fecal matter, viruses, an acute imbalance of intestinal bacteria, unfamiliar foods and food intolerance, allergies, attacks of external bacteria (such as cholera, typhoid, or bacillary dysentery), eating unripe fruit or tainted food or water, emotional turmoil (such as fear, nervousness, or rage), or infestation of parasites such as worms or amoebas (as in amoebic dysentery).

Autopsy of an impacted colon taken from the above patient, after death.

98

Diarrhea may even be a symptom of cancer. If the stools are black or there is blood in them, one should immediately seek a doctor.

People suffer from diarrhea quite frequently in our culture. There are many reasons people get diarrhea, but the most common is constipation.

So many times, clients complain of constipation, then diarrhea, then again constipation, followed by diarrhea.

What happens is the colon has so much impaction that the colon muscles cannot expel the feces. The body senses this irritation in attempts to remove the impaction. It washes it with fluid, causing diarrhea, which is the liquid form that expels out of the colon. As a result, stool becomes hard as a rock, tearing delicate tissues and creating a hemorrhoid.

Testimonial

Diverticulitis Symptoms Gone

Dear Millan:
My sister and my mother both recommended your colonics.
After doing the cleansing program, I noticed I didn't have the symptoms of diverticulitis anymore. What a relief to not have to rush to the bathroom and not make it.
Thank you so much.

Signed,
Jan M.

Irritable Bowel Syndrome

Gastroenterologists cite irritable bowel syndrome as the most common aliment. Symptoms of this frustrating and painful condition are abdominal pain (only temporarily relieved by frequent bowel movements), a bloated or distended abdomen, and mucus in the stools. Rectal bleeding is not a trademark of this condition.

Irritable bowel syndrome is brought on by a variety of causes, including nervousness and anxiety, unfamiliar food, too spicy food, food allergies and intolerance, and, of course, bad diet.

Testimonial

A Relief from Irritable Bowel Syndrome

Dear Millan:
I've always had the symptoms of Irritable Bowel Syndrome. The frequency and intensity of pain grew as I grew, and by the time I was 19 years old it was happening once every two weeks, the pain being so intense my only focus was to lay on my back on the floor, and try to breathe, and pray I would get through just one more time, for about 5 to 15 minutes and it would vanish.

I went to doctors, but they would just say "fecal impaction" and give me a harsh laxative and send me on my way. During my attacks I would never vomit or have a bowel movement but I used the laxatives the doctors gave me and would be shaky and tired for a few days after, but then I would feel a lot better for a week or so, so I thought this was ok. That all changed. I would have the attacks now for more like 30 minutes. I was in so much pain my body was pale and sweaty but cold and weak. I could barely speak to ask to be taken to the emergency room because I could barely breathe without a stab of pain.

In my 4 days and 3 nights at the hospital, I endured drinking a gallon of salty water to completely empty my system; afterwards I was dizzy and could barely move. Then I was given a colonoscopy. I was told my white blood cell count was excessively high, and I was given antibiotics. This is when I found out I have Irritable Bowel Syndrome. The doctor said it was just a genetic thing you are born with and you have to deal with it your whole life. Apparently, that particular time, I had gotten a bit of bad bacteria somehow and it

100

settled in my colon, turning my Irritable Bowel Syndrome into Ischemic Colitis (an infection in the lining of the colon). When I left the hospital the doctor basically said, 'We have no idea why this happens, the only thing we can do is give you a prescription for pain killers and anti-spasmodic, so that when it does happen, you can soften the blow with the drugs, oh and eat a low residue diet for a few weeks, then go to high fiber foods. BYE!!!' That's when I decided to start learning about my body, health, nutrition, and exercise.

I started eating high fiber foods, drinking 64 oz. of water a day and working out. Then God stepped in; I heard about Millan and her work. I am thankful to say that since I started the cleansing sessions, I haven't had one attack. Thank God. I feel healthier and I have more energy. I know nutrition and exercise play a big role and staying healthy, but for me so has the colon hydrotherapy.

Signed, Angela C.

Inflammatory Bowel Disease

Resembling irritable bowel syndrome is inflammatory bowel disease. But the latter's cause is a serious imbalance of intestinal flora. The toxins given off by suddenly proliferating "bad bacteria" irritate and inflame the lining of the bowel and may cause ulceration or perforation of the delicate colon wall.

Obviously, an impacted, constipated colon can be deadly in this case. Unhealthy diet and a stagnating colon are to blame.

This disease continues to subvert conventional views of the importance of diet in the colon and overall health. A more complete discussion of this condition can be found in Galland's and Barrie's report, "Intestinal Dysbiosis and the Causes of Disease," cited earlier in this book and available from the Great Smokies Diagnostic Laboratory in Asheville, N. Carolina.

101

Ulcerative Colitis
Ulcerative colitis is an inflammation of the lining of the colon, with possible complications due to perforation of the wall. Again, it is the product of bad diet, improper colon function, and bowel habits.

Crohn's Disease
Crohn's disease is a different kind of inflammation that can occur anywhere in the digestive tract from the mouth to the rectum, but characteristically it is found in the lower bowel. The inflammation attacks the entire wall of the colon, not just its interior lining.

Dr. Henry Janowitz has noted that people who suffer from these inflammatory diseases have depressed immune systems. He suspects that the decreased immune response may be a direct result of the disease and not the cause.

Testimonial

Victim of Crohn's Disease

Dear Millan:
I was diagnosed with Crohn's disease. I went through years of pain and took all medications required. I then had surgery. It returned 1 year later with chronic diarrhea.

I then started your cleansing program. The cleansing program included diet change. This has eliminated all symptoms of the Crohn's disease. I feel so much better now.

The bonus to this story is that I lost 20 pounds!!!!Thank you so much,
Trish

Diverticulosis/Diverticulitis
Diverticulosis is a condition in which abnormal diverticula (sac-like pouches) develop on the walls of the digestive tract. Most are found on the colon.

This condition is caused by impacted fecal matter. When the pouches become inflamed, the condition is known as diverticulitis. The irritation can be severe, in some cases perforating the colon, necessitating surgery.

The constant irritation and drain on the immune system is an invitation to cancer.

This condition is more common in civilized society, with high-meat, low-fiber diets. It is especially dangerous in the elderly. It is well documented that the lowest incidents of diverticulitis in our society is among the Seventh-Day Adventists, due to their lifestyle, including a vegetarian diet.

Jaw and Dental Ailments
Some forms of TMJ (temporomandibular joint syndrome) are particularly mysterious and unbearably painful to its sufferers. Clients with this condition have stated that internal cleansing and dietary cleansing have helped to control inflammation of the jaw area.

Other forms of oral maladies have been responsive to internal cleansing, as this case indicates:

Testimonial

Painful Mouth Condition

For a year, I suffered an extremely painful condition that made sores in my mouth. The pain was constant and so great that my whole jawbone area swelled visibly. I took aspirin regularly, but it did not help. My dentist recommended I see a specialist, since nothing he tried worked. But the specialist could not help me either. All he recommended was surgery, and warned me I might have cancer.

Desperate, I tried internal cleansing. After a few sessions, to my relief, the pain went away completely, and I have had the first pain-free week in over a year.

Recently I went back to my doctor and told him of my experience with internal cleansing. He said, "What's that?"

All the anticipation of possible surgery and fear of cancer are now behind me. I am very grateful.

Signed
Walter

CHAPTER SEVEN

Quote: You are awesomely made in his image. I will help you keep it that way.
Millan Chessman

TOXINS

Authorities in the health field agree: toxins and poisons in the body stem from a toxic bowel. Remember, just because you have not taken social drugs or medications does not mean your body is not toxic.

When someone asks, "How do I know I have a toxic condition? I am healthy as a horse," I reply a typical Western diet consisting of too much meat, pasteurized, homogenized dairy, processed food, and refined sugar guarantees toxicity.

Sooner or later, the price for violating your body must be paid. Maybe not today or tomorrow, but the time will come.

I guarantee it.

Cleansing the body eliminates blockages, dead cells, toxins, poisons, excess mucus, environmental pollutants, and greatly improves circulation. Our bodies are now hazardous waste dumps when you realize that the average American consumes one pound of food additives per year! "Monosodium glutamate, sugar substitutes, dyes, preservatives (including nitrates), emulsifiers, fillers, waxes, tenderizers, texturizers, antifreezes, synthetics, genetically engineered foods, hormones and antibiotics are just a few of the chemicals added to a wide variety of processed foods. Tens of thousands of people have had adverse reactions, including death, to certain food chemical preservatives. Over 3,000 chemical food additives hide in our food" (Vegetarian Times).

The Atlanta based Centers for Disease Control and Prevention (CDC) estimates that Americans suffer at least 325,000 annual cases food borne illnesses from fish. If you eat a shucked oyster, you're eating its intestines in a raw form. One study reviewed by the CDC and Doug Archer, Ph.D., shows that fish with fins are less likely to cause food borne disease compared to fish, beef or poultry (although shellfish is far more dangerous than either). Isn't that an interesting scientific fact? In the Bible, God commanded His people to eat only the fish with fins and scales.

Producers of the *Prime Time Live* ABC TV program enlisted "Longo" to play the part of a typical consumer, sending her off to buy about fifty pounds of fish from markets in New York, Boston, Chicago and Baltimore. Then, the fish were tested in the laboratories for contamination. Twenty percent had harmful bacteria levels - higher than would be safe for humans to eat. About forty percent of them contained human fecal matter at a higher level than anyone should consume.

An EPA study published in 1992 found DDE, a chemical resulting from the breakdown of the pesticide DDT, in more than 98% of 388 freshwater sites. DDT was banned in 1973, yet it is still appearing on plates of seafood! Several other hazardous chemicals, PCBs and Mercury for example, turned up in more than 90% of the site samples.

The following information on toxins comes from excerpts of an article entitled, "Hidden Dangers in Your Food and Water" in an issue of *McCall's Magazine.*

Cell biologist Ana Soto, M.D., was perplexed. The breast-cancer cells she was working with in the laboratory were supposed to thrive only when 'fed' the female hormone es-

106

trogen. But the cells were growing without added estrogen. After months of puzzlement, Soto found the cancer cells' secret hormone source. The plastic equipment used in her experiment, it seemed, was releasing an estrogen-like chemical into the cell culture, causing the cancer cells to grow.

"Our environment contains many manmade chemicals that may alter the effects of natural estrogen when they enter the human body in food and water," explains Terri Damstra, a toxicologist.

Here are some of the chemicals that may mimic or block estrogen in the body:

DDT and its breakdown product, DDE: DDT is now banned in the United States, but is still present in our environment.

Polychlorinated Biphenyls (PCBs): These industrial compounds have been restricted in the United States but will linger in our environment for decades to come.

Dioxins: These chemical compounds - often produced during garbage incineration or as a result of paper bleaching - can be released into the air, water and soil.

Experts point to the example of the now infamous pregnancy drug diethylstilbestrol (DES). This drug, used between 1940 and 1971, was a powerful synthetic estrogen designed to prevent miscarriages. Its use resulted in a high rate of cancer and reproductive problems in both the women who took the drug and their offspring.

Women, having a greater percentage of body fat than men, can accumulate a heavy burden of these toxins, especially in fatty tissues such as the breasts. Laboratory studies at NIEHS show that inside the body, environmental estrogens can bind to estrogen receptors on a cell's surface and either mimic or block the effects of natural estrogen. 'We have to be careful about how we interpret these

107

studies,' says Sandra Eirey of the Chemical Manufacturers Association (CMA). Several studies found that women with breast cancer tended to have higher concentrations of the organochlorines DDT, DDE or PCBs in their fat tissue than did other women.

Some evidence suggests that estrogenic and antiestrogenic pollutants can endanger developing fetuses. Other experts suspect that fetal exposure to dioxins may be responsible for a significant drop in sperm counts since 1940, which has been documented in the U.S. and in many other countries. In a single meal, a person may get PCBs in the fish and pesticides on the vegetables.

I believe there is an urgency to cleanse our bodies in this polluted environment we are living in! Internal cleansing is the number one solution to ridding our bodies of the buildup of these toxic chemicals.

Mercury Toxins

Today, some dentists are removing amalgams (mercury fillings) from teeth. This is important to our body's well-being and a detoxified body. Yet, because their bodies are autointoxicated, patients are not getting the full benefit of this procedure.

In Sweden, Dr. Crister Inged Malmstromon studied patients who had mercury amalgams removed. Interestingly, the subjects had not recovered from the symptoms of mercury toxicity.

Only after undergoing a detoxification program of internal cleansing were the poisons released.

Laboratory examinations on fecal matter removed during internal cleansing showed mercury toxins in old stool lodged in colon pockets. Following the cleansings, patients actually recovered from the mercury toxicity.

Another study discovered eighty-five percent of mercury toxins leave the body via the colon. In other words, an improperly functioning colon hinders mercury from passing. Ultimately, mercury implanted on colon walls absorbs back into the body.

An internal cleansing program is essential to the full recovery of a mercury-toxified body.

Amalgam removal is expensive; moreover, it does not thoroughly cleanse the body from toxins. Internal cleansing is relatively inexpensive, ranging from fifty dollars to one hundred dollars a session.

David Louis, in 2001 *Fascinating Facts*, states:

Undertakers report that human bodies do not deteriorate as quickly as they used to. The reason for this, they believe, is that the modern diet contains so many preservatives that these chemicals tend to prevent the body from decomposing too rapidly after.

Tell me we do not need to cleanse our bodies. It was told to me by a military doctor that during the Vietnam War, the bodies of the American soldiers decomposed very slowly in comparison to the bodies of the Vietnamese soldiers.

Autointoxication

Basically, we poison our bodies with our forks by eating the wrong foods as well as overeating. Remember, our bodies were never designed to handle flesh food.

Why do we bathe every day, brush our teeth, gargle with mouthwash, and pour on the perfume? We are trying to camouflage the smell of sewage inside our bodies.

This is chronic autointoxication.

This condition factors into most chronic disorders. Millions of putrefactive bacteria fill the flesh of dead animals.

I am proud of my grown-up granddaughter, Lareesa. She has not eaten any kind of flesh food since she was eight years old.

She says, "Grammy, I just love animals too much to eat them."

People are poisoning themselves from the inside out (known as autointoxication or autotoxemia). Brought on by a body desperately trying to defend itself against disease, this condition is an invitation to a weakened immune system for viral and bacterial attack, vulnerability to allergens, and hormonal and other chemical imbalances. The body will excrete offensive odors as it tries to eliminate accumulated sewage through pores and other body areas (like the mouth, ears, nose, groin, armpits, and vagina).

It is not an attractive state!

Other symptoms of toxicity are unexplained: weakness, fatigue, listlessness, lethargy, or sluggishness, inability to focus or concentrate, confusion, "spaciness," apathy, depression, unexplained mood swings, irritability, or chronic, unexplained anxiety.

Testimonial

Agent Orange Removed

Dear Millan:

I was in Vietnam November 1966 to November 1967. They dumped Agent Orange on us on a regular basis. Agent Orange is toxic and fatal. We saw the yellow clouds as they came down. It was used to kill the foliage in order to see the enemy.

I discovered by my tenth series of colonics in 1997 that I was eliminating the same yellow toxins from Agent Orange from 31 years ago, at long last. I eliminated about 51 flushes of yellow toxins and I feel like my liver is better now.

My lungs and liver became very clear because of the colonics.

Thank You,
Larry M.

110

Doctors Discuss Autotoxemia

Fifty-seven prominent British physicians met in London to discuss the problem of autointoxication (or autotoxemia).

These eminent doctors determined the major cause of autotoxemia to be an inefficient, "toxic" colon. They identified twenty-two poisons originating from an unhealthy colon. Among them is a chilling array of lethal toxins, including: cadaverine, cresol, botulin, putrescine, ammonia, methylmercaptam, methylgardinine, sulfuroglovbine, sulfuretted hydrogen, hydrogen sulfide, sepsis, hydrogen, indole, phenol, nitric acid, urobilin, histidine, muscarine, indican, neurin, ptomaine, pentemethylendiamine, and indoethylamine.

These toxic chemicals also kill the genuinely beneficial microorganisms - lactobacillus acidophilus and bifidus bacteria - enabling the marginally beneficial smaller colony of E. coli II to thrive and multiply out of control, spewing ever more deadly poisons into our bloodstream and tissues.

Is it any wonder that our bodies get sick in all possible ways? Toxicity in its raw form outside our bodies does not change its toxic effects when cycled throughout our bodies. We allow our colon to become clogged with toxins through poor diet and lifestyle, bad toilet training, medical and scientific ignorance, and culturally mandated indifference. Many poisons stay inside our bodies for a lifetime. This toxicity causes illness and a rundown immune system. I believe that autointoxication left untreated ages us.

Testimonial

Toxins & Sickness Gone

Dear Millan:
My experience at your clinic has been a wonderful healing and learning time in my life. After being sick and never feeling very well, I was

---

toxic. Cleansing was the best decision I've ever made.

I look and feel much better and I don't get sick anymore. My life has changed for the better and I will continue the principles. In fact, I'm so happy about my health I am telling others so they can get healthy too.

Anonymous

Autotoxemia: Researchers' Findings

The concept of autotoxemia was first articulated late in the last century by the eminent Russian bacteriologist, Metchnikoff. At the time, his discoveries were revolutionary because of their newness and far-ranging implications.

This was an age that was just beginning to see through more powerful and accurate microscopes the reality of bacteria and understand their prevalence and significance in the world.

The implications Metchnikoff theorized for these microorganisms were largely ignored in the United States. Yet, they influenced four generations of European physicians as far as bowel functions and overall health is concerned.

Metchnikoff believed that autotoxemia (self-poisoning) through putrefaction of metabolic wastes in the large intestine is the main cause of preventable illness and premature aging.

Recently, Drs. Leo Galland, Senior Research Consultant of the Great Smokies Diagnostic Laboratory in Ashville, North Carolina, and Stephen Barrie, the laboratory's president, released their findings on autotoxemia in a paper called "Intestinal Dysbiosis and the Causes of Disease."

It is only in the last two decades, with the frightening rise in colorectal cancer, that Metchnikoff's ideas have been taken seriously here in the United States. Finally, serious research has begun on the relationship between our health - with emphasis on the colon - and what we eat.

Galland and Barrie's research "has implicated bacterial dysbiosis in a number of inflamma-

112

tions within the bowel or involving skin or connective tissue," such as atopic eczema, irritable bowel syndrome, and inflammatory bowel disease. The researchers further note the following:

> *Immunologic responses to gut flora have been advanced by several authors as important factors in the pathogenesis of inflammatory joint diseases. It is well known that reactive arthritis can be activated by intestinal infections with... enterobacteria... Increased intestinal permeability and immune responses to bacterial debris may cause other types of inflammatory joint diseases as well.*

The researchers at the Great Smokies Laboratory found that "most adverse effects of the indigenous gut flora are caused by the intense metabolic activity" of bacteria mainly concerned with the waste products of food.

They continue:

> *The enzymes urease, found [in these organisms] and induced in [them] by a diet high in meat, hydrolyses [or transforms] urea to ammonia, raising stool pH. A relatively high stool pH is associated with a higher prevalence of colon cancer.*

Conversely, the researchers state, "a relatively low stool pH is associated with protection against colon cancer."

They also found that "bacterial tryptophanase degrades tryptophan to carcinogenic phenols and like urease, is induced by a high flesh food diet." An American diet, typically high in flesh food, is the major culprit in colorectal cancer. It is also receiving attention for its contributing factors to breast cancer.

Galland and Barrie have more to say on the dangers of cancer-causing toxins in a clogged colon:

> *Bile acids irritate the colon's delicate lining and cause diarrhea. Moreover, bile acids or their metabolites [byproducts] appear to be carcinogenic and are thought to con-*

113

tribute to the development of colon cancer and to ulcerative colitis.

To further complicate a dangerous situation, gut bacteria are more likely to contribute to colon carcinogenesis (beginnings of cancer conditions in cells, or protocancers); in fact, the prevalence of colon cancer is proportional to stool concentration of a particulate secondary bile acid."

The researchers go on to state that these disturbances are caused by the high fat, flesh and depleted fiber content, which characterizes Western diets and are consistent with Metchnikoff's theories.

The obvious answer for patients with chronic gastrointestinal, inflammatory or autoimmune disorders, food allergy, intolerance, breast and colon cancer, and unexplained fatigue, malnutrition or neuropsychiatric symptoms, is to eliminate and prevent further disorders through internal cleansing, along with a plant-based diet.

CHAPTER EIGHT

WHY CLEANSE

Blocked Colons
The colon builds up blockage just like the plumbing at home or the corrosive build-up in a car's engine.

People have many pounds of waste in the colon! Autopsies I have witnessed confirm this to be true.

If you are driving your car and the red light on your dash indicates there is a problem, do you ignore the warning and keep going as though the problem doesn't exist?

Of course not.

Yet we do the same to our bodies until we feel a pain or ache. Then we go to the doctor's office and get a prescription to mask the pain.

We seldom go further to get to the real cause and not just treat the symptoms. Our body parts are so interconnected. When one hurts, one should consider cleaning out the colon and detoxifying the system. The body will hurt because it is in a state of autointoxication.

Your body cannot assimilate nutrients if it is toxic. It is that simple.

We buy hundreds of vitamins and minerals and expect to feel better—yet often we do not. Then we wonder why.

A client must clean out the body and then add the nutrition. See and feel the difference.

Some clients say, "Gee, what is wrong? Why don't I feel better?"

115

They change their diets and eat nutritious foods. They virtually cut out meat, dairy, and processed foods. They start exercise programs and take the best vitamins and minerals money can buy.

Yet why do they not feel better?

They must clean out their systems! There are many reasons we are unhealthy: a poor diet, a toxic system, lack of exercise, heredity, and environment. A severely impacted colon can press painfully against the diaphragm and cause breathing problems, as my client Clyde's story demonstrates:

Testimonial

Client Finds Relief from Impacted Colon
I used to have tightness near my rib cage and had problems breathing. I went to the doctor and he said nothing was wrong, I just needed to lose weight. My whole abdomen felt full. A series of internal cleansing sessions moved this blockage and the tightness disappeared. I have not had that tightness since and it has been a year.

Signed
Clyde

Suppressed Emotions - Suppressed Bowel
In my experience, I have observed women to have more digestive problems than men, especially in the colon area. I believe women have a tendency to hold their feelings inside and suppress them. These emotions go right to the digestive system and hinder the bowel from proper action.

Men have a tendency to be more expressive and less emotional; therefore, they have more bowel movements than women, on the average.

Interestingly, my clientele is pretty much fifty-fifty men and women.

I might add, the frequency of men's bowel movements does not necessarily mean women are more toxic than men. Just because men's bowels

116

move daily does not mean their bodies are clean and their colons are completely evacuated.

Such an assumption has been disproved time and time again.

In primitive areas of the world, constipation is unheard of. In fact, people living in small communities, farms, and ranches have fewer digestive problems overall. Those living in the civilized world, experience higher blood pressure, allergies, diabetes, arthritis, constipation, asthma - the list goes on and on.

And those of us in the field of health know this all stems primarily from unhealthy diets and toxic bowels.

We need to clean out our colon.

Four Steps to Good Health
There are four steps to good health.

First, it would be ideal if humans could exclusively eat vegetables, fruits, grains, legumes, raw nuts, and seeds. I know this must seem like an impossible objective for most, but the closer one comes to it, the better one feels.

Second, cleanse the body.

Third, exercise, whether it be walking, aerobics, bike-riding, etc. Break a sweat.

Fourth, a daily intake of good vitamins and minerals is essential because many nutrients are lacking in so many foods. I recommend a quality barley powder product and to eat organic foods.

Also, an important factor is fasting. I recommend a 24-48 hour green smoothie or water fast once a week on a regular basis for optimum health. There's an easy way to accomplish this without much discomfort. On the first day, eat your big meal around noon, until your stomach is comfortably full. That evening make a green smoothie or have hot vegetable broth. The next morning, drink hot decaf herbal tea, organic coffee or fruit smoothie. I do this myself and it keeps my weight in check.

117

A Look Inside the Body

There is a documented case of the death of a thirty-eight year-old man. When his colon was examined, it was 19 inches in diameter and weighed almost one hundred pounds. In contrast, a normal colon is 2 to 2 1/2 inches in diameter.

Look around at many of the people with potbellies. Granted, fat is there, but also pocketed in the colon are pounds of old, impacted stool.

The danger occurs when impacted stool bursts through colon walls and the walls become infected – this is when diverticulitis results. This is a very common condition; moreover, it is evident that half of my clients suffer from hemorrhoids.

In his book, Dr. Norman Walker writes about a young epileptic patient. Walker recommended six weeks of internal cleansing for the girl. After the fifth week, there were no visible results, and the patient's family became discouraged. Finally, after the end of the fifth week, lo and behold, this young lady passed a fist-full of worms during her session.

After that, she never had another epileptic seizure.

Years of abuse to our bodies cannot be remedied overnight. We live in a society of instant results, yet obtaining good health just does not work that way.

Women with prolapsed, transverse colons (from my research, seventy percent of people in the western world have prolapsed colons) are likely to have some female problems: positive Pap smears, vaginal infections, discharge, and so forth.

A normal-looking colon is very rare. Most X-rays show twisted, looped, and ballooned colons.

Why?

Because of diet.

We eat very little fiber foods and way too much of the wrong foods. One time, a nurse told me she watched a doctor perform colon surgery.

The surgeon observed feces in the patient's colon and just sewed it back up, leaving the fecal matter right where it was.

Testimonial

A sufferer of Asthma and Allergies

Dear Millan: For the last 12 years, I have suffered from allergies, chronic sinusitis, and severe asthma. I have undergone surgery two times to correct the sinus problems only to return to the same (if not more severe) condition in a matter of months. I have been hospitalized twice with pneumonia. By the time I came to see you, I was taking high doses of Prednisone (an oral steroid), Theodur, and albuterol inhalers.

I was very much overweight and my eating habits were terrible. You gave me a cleansing diet to follow, taking careful note to eliminate all the mucous causing foods such as white sugar, white flour, and meats (including poultry and fish). I was told to eat a diet rich in fresh fruit and vegetables, whole grains and fresh juices, and I was started on a series of colonics.

After just two weeks, I was able to wean myself off of Prednisone, and Theodur completely and have not been on these oral medications. I was also able to reduce the use of my inhalers. About this time, I noticed that my sinuses began draining and my nose ran for about the next three to four weeks straight! By the sixth to seventh week of my cleanse, my sinuses had cleared up completely and my sense of smell had returned! My allergies were gone and my sneezing stopped! I read that parasites are involved in 100% of asthma cases and I was anxious to begin the Parasite Cleanse in the eighth week of my cleansing program. It was not easy but I was determined to see it through. During the week, I was taking the parasite cleansing herbs. I experienced some asthma type reactions and coughing.

119

I also experienced some pain in my back and occasional sharp twinges of pain in my lungs. However, after being off of the herbs for about one week, one day I experienced a quick return to easy breathing and felt better than I ever had before. That day I went for a nice, brisk, 45-minute walk with my husband. Later that afternoon I passed what appeared to be flukes and a 2-foot long white-colored worm! A couple of weeks later, I repeated the parasite cleanse, a little more comfortable this time.

My lungs seemed to be clearing themselves out again and I had a great deal of productive coughing. Again, I passed more worms.

Your colonics and cleansing program contributed to the complete recovery I have experienced

Thank you,
Michelle

Influences on Regularity

Pleasurable emotions and excitement that one may experience can positively affect the colon towards elimination. On the other hand, depression, despondency, anger, desire for revenge, bitterness, and stress can halt the functioning of the digestive system and cause constipation. Animal and human studies have proven this.

Exercise is very important in keeping the colon healthy. I know a person who jumps on the trampoline daily to move her bowels. And it works! She swears by it and recommends it to others.

When one sits a lot, the colon muscles do not function properly. Many clients are truck drivers or airplane pilots who sit for long periods and are not able to go to the bathroom when the urge hits them.

Posture has been mentioned repeatedly among health authorities and cannot be emphasized enough; it is vital to the proper functioning of the colon.

Be aware of how you are standing. Are your shoulders back? Is your chest out? Is your head up high?

How about when you are sitting? Are you straight up? Is your chin up? You will find that correct posture greatly aids in bowel elimination.

Testimonial

Reinvigorated Emotions

Dear Millan:
Before I came to your clinic, I suffered from severe anxiety and fear. Not only was I fatigued, but I was also depressed. During this time, I had absolutely no appetite, and my menstrual cycle had stopped completely. On top of it all, I experienced horrible headaches, and even discovered that my body contained worms.

After I went through a series of cleanses at your clinic my situation made a quick turnaround.

I now have more mental alertness, less anxiety, less fatigue and depression. My appetite greatly increased, and my period came after three months.

Thank you so very much for all of your wonderful services.

Sincerely,
Xochtl

When my clients cleanse the inside of their bodies for the first time, they notice a difference in body odor and skin. Their breath is naturally fresh, recalling the sweet wine, apples, or peaches romantic poets rhapsodized about in their sonnets of passion and love. A client can wear colognes or perfumes simply because the smell is pleasing, not because of a need to cover up foul odor.

121

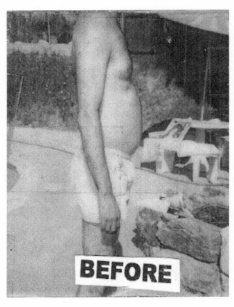

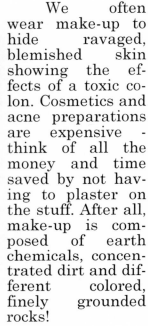

We often wear make-up to hide ravaged, blemished skin showing the effects of a toxic colon. Cosmetics and acne preparations are expensive - think of all the money and time saved by not having to plaster on the stuff. After all, make-up is composed of earth chemicals, concentrated dirt and different colored, finely grounded rocks!

After internal cleansing, this client's waistline and stomach size were reduced.

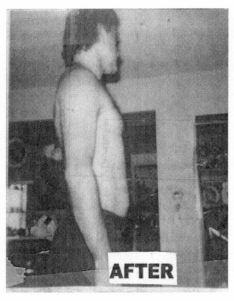

Testimonial

Looks Younger & Bloating Gone

Dear Millan:

I have been having health problems for the last nine months with diarrhea and constipation. On my honeymoon, anytime I ate, I had diarrhea. It was to the point that when my husband barely touched my stomach, I had severe pain. I tried taking psyllium and that did not work. If I ate cheese, I would get severe pain.

I had to take time off work and ended up in the emergency room. If I went outside or slept with the window open, I would become very ill. I would have flu like symptoms. This went on for years.

I started on your cleansing program and now my husband says my body odor is gone and all of the liver spots on my face have disappeared. This cleansing has made me look younger.

I have lost weight and all of the above symptoms have disappeared. I go to the bathroom regularly and no longer experienced pain in my stomach. I now do not catch everything that goes around and sleep with my window open.

Now my husband chases me around the house.

I eat no more flesh foods or cheese and I am a new person.

Sincerely, Regina

Attentive care of the colon is important education, just as important as valuing lungs for breathing, hearts for circulation, blood for distributing oxygen and nutrients to every cell, genitals for sexual pleasure, and brains for intellect, mind, imagination, and soul.

Try as we might to avoid the subject, there is no getting around the fact that digestion includes elimination.

All other processes depend on correctly functioning kidneys and a healthy colon. People die if they cannot eliminate urine or fecal matter. Today, people typically defecate once a day instead

123

of a minimum of three times daily, as they really should. Healthy elimination is defecation after each meal. True, urine and feces present possible contamination with disease bacteria and other pathogens; however, it is important to note that poor diet or medication in the system cause urine and feces to be odoriferous.

Victory over PMS
Think you have premenstrual syndrome? It could be, but some symptoms are very similar to a simply unhealthy colon crying out desperately for help.

Testimonial
20 Pounds of Excess Waste

Dear Millan:
Before, my abdomen hurt, and it was very bloated. I suffered from chronic fatigue and indigestion. My hair was thin, skin was dry and kept breaking out, and menstruation was irregular. I was carrying twenty pounds of excess weight. My thinking was fuzzy, and I had a hard time concentrating. I was weak and short of breath, and I only urinated one to two times a day. My bowels consisted of diarrhea and then constipation. I was not digesting foods; whole pieces came out. I could not sweat, and could not work or hold a job. In addition, I had goiters and candidiasis. After internal cleansing: I had tremendous energy.
Now I enjoy swimming and roller-blading, and my digestion is good. My skin is clear and soft, and my hair is thicker than ever before in my whole life. Menstruation is back to normal, and goiters are gone. Water weight is gone, as well as the candidiasis. My thought processes are great: I am in school and working.
In fact, I started my own business. As depressed as I was before, now I am very happy. Even my bad breath is gone.
SignedSusan

124

Women's Female Problems

For women, sometimes uncomfortable or even painful sexual intercourse, persistent unexplained vaginal odor, chronic or recurring yeast infections, and PMS, are symptoms of toxicity and an impacted colon.

Testimonial

Libido Booster

I was a meat eater all of my life. At the age of forty, I began to notice that I would get an erection, but after a few minutes, it would diminish. This was a major problem with my sexual relationship with my wife. I blamed it on being tired or stressed.

After reading about vegetarianism, I decided to eliminate all animal products from my diet and cleanse. Lo and behold, exactly six months later I realized that my libido changed. I no longer needed to use Viagra. I was able to get an erection, sustain it. I attribute my success to the colonics I had and the fact that I stopped eating white flour, white sugar, pasteurized homogenized dairy, and processed foods. Now I eat fruits, vegetables, grains, legumes, raw nuts, and seeds.

Ralph

Sexual Dysfunction

Too many women suffer unnecessary sexual dysfunction. When no physical causes are discovered, a woman is usually advised to get psychological help or go to a sex or marriage counselor. This is humiliating when the real problem is not subconscious resistance, revulsion, or lack of technique, but could possibly be the result of an impacted colon.

125

Modern medicine is so compartmentalized by specialty that bowel problems remain largely invisible, and may even be entirely misdiagnosed as other problems

But what a difference internal cleansing made in one woman's sex life! This woman was diagnosed with a tipped uterus, which was accurate, but her uterus was tipped because her over-full colon was leaning on it. The doctors missed the impacted colon in every case. As she tells it:

Testimonial

Painful Sex

Prior to internal cleansing, doctors told me my uterus was tipped. I had constant pain in the right and lower left abdominal area.

During sexual intercourse, I felt pain in the back of my cervix. My husband said he could feel the wall inside the vagina. Because of my great discomfort and pain, he had to be careful.

After I began the dietary cleansing program with the series of internal cleansing, my husband remarked that he could not feel the pressure of the back wall with his penis anymore. And I no longer had pain during intercourse.

My relationship with my husband is far more enjoyable because the pain is gone. I no longer have to cry out for him to stop.

Anonymous

Substitute Aphrodisiacs

Cologne and perfume were invented originally as a means of masking the turn-off of a dirty body's odors and because the scents were pleasant, it made them a good substitute aphrodisiac. Colognes, perfumes, and even alcoholic beverages were used for millennia to sweeten fetid breath from a dirty, decaying mouth, pungent meals, and bad digestion. Today, for the same reasons, we keep the makers of breath fresheners rolling in greenbacks and coins!

Brushing your teeth and performing optimal oral hygiene, bathing, or showering daily are good, practical, refreshing, and disease preventing activities. We know today the health benefits of a clean body, clean hands and a clean mouth. But when was the last time you bathed the inside of your body (where all the smell really originates) and honestly considered your diet and exercise level?

Testimonial

Recovery from Herpes

I have had an active herpes condition for about nineteen years. As I get older, I break out more times each month.

Since I have started this cleansing program, I have not had any new lesions, and that has been now ten weeks. What a blessing

Signed,
Mildred

Body Hygiene and Internal Cleansing

Because we work and live closely together in offices, exercise gyms, cars, buses, theaters, restaurants, and homes, we are naturally concerned about our body hygiene.

For better or worse, our appearance and personal odor influence how we are perceived by our employers, co-workers, people we do business with, friends, lovers, and family members. Even those people with whom we pray and worship are not immune from the impressions of their senses.

The primary origin of offensive smells emanating from our bodies - such as strong body odor and bad breath - is a toxic body and sluggish colon.

Testimonial

Embarrassing Body Odor Problem

Dear Millan:
    I want to thank you for the series of colonics I received from you. They helped me so much. I had embarrassing body odor problems and recurring dirty earwax. Now, both problems are gone and there are other benefits.

Thanks again, HN

CHAPTER NINE

Quote: Defeat is a stepping stone to victory and success. Millan Chessman

SOLUTION TO AN UNHEALTHY DIET

Colon hydrotherapy, in conjunction with the herbal cleansing program and juice fast or modified diet, successfully eliminates old mucoid fecal matter.

This is one of the benefits of internal cleansing; it effectively removes any entrenched mucoid fecal matter as far up the colon as the cecum (the beginning of the large intestine, where the water meets the ileocecal valve) and the small intestine.

Internal cleansing eliminates the toxins trapped and recycled by a sluggish colon.

Since a sluggish colon prevents proper elimination of metabolic waste by the liver and kidneys (which usually filters out poisons), this waste is reabsorbed into the bloodstream and lymphatic system. The influx of recycled waste, therefore, overworks the liver and kidneys.

Cleansing the colon, in combination with a good diet, exercise, and plenty of pure fluids, helps prevent the absorption of toxins that would otherwise enter the bloodstream through the colon wall.

A clean colon reduces the colon wall's exposure to carcinogens.

A clean colon is vital in preventive medicine because it establishes a healthy internal environment.

A clean colon improves and strengthens the immune system. A hydrated body improves lymph flow. Once this is done, the body's natural immune responses to numerous illnesses are boosted.

With a healthy, intact immune system, my clients are not debilitated by weakness and fatigue as their bodies try unsuccessfully to thwart disease. Instead, they get the benefit of renewed energy and zest for life.

Therapy Stimulates Peristalsis

Colon hydrotherapy stimulates the natural mechanical action of a sluggish or "flaccid" colon to resume normal peristalsis. Colon hydrotherapy helps to tone up and exercise the colon so it can begin to take care of itself. When the large intestine is flaccid and holding mucoidal fecal matter, it cannot contract effectively. The blood supply is inhibited. Little beneficial absorption or waste elimination can happen.

When the sewage is cleaned out of the colon, it can begin to function efficiently again, which causes the blood supply and its vital transference functions to improve. This, in turn, improves water and mineral absorption.

Testimonial

Less Cellulite, No Body Odor, and Healthier Skin

Since my internal cleansing, I have noticed my cellulite has diminished, and my skin has gotten softer!

Before, my skin was chalky and dull. I have lost four pounds, which is great, and my skin appears healthier.

What impressed me the most was I no longer have body odor under my arms the way I used to.

People have commented that my skin looks great. I feel very good.

Signed,
Cookie

Fresh-Scented People

The profits of the multi-billion dollar cosmetic, deodorant, and perfume industries testify to our obsession with looking beautiful and smelling "as fresh as spring flowers."

A clean colon permits clean, natural body odors to exude from our bodies. We are a society of cleanliness and hygiene, yet we walk around with worms, parasites, and sewage in our bodies. We use perfumes and deodorant to camouflage body odors coming from within.

My clients have claimed that when their body is internally clean, it is not necessary to bathe daily. Did you know that your breath could be sweet smelling without having to brush your teeth every day?

Did you know that the smell God intended for your body is the most pleasant odor you can imagine?

One man shared that he had been living with a woman for a few years. He said her vagina smelled so bad he could not have sex with her. He told her so, and she went to the doctor for help. The doctor told her he could not do anything for her. He stated that was just the way her body was functioning.

How pathetic. This problem could have been resolved. There are many reported cases where sexual relationships improved through the colon-cleansing program.

Testimonial

Cleansing Saved my Life

Dear Millan:

I have recommended the cleansing program to several. I have also mailed your book to my son in Houston, Texas. I believe this cleansing program saved my life. I believe it is a good program for everyone.

Thank you, Millan!

Signed, Lucille

131

No More Potbelly!

My clients have commented on their tummies being flatter due to internal cleansing. Much of that potbelly is the result of an ill-toned colon. Even after years of rigorous dieting and exhausting strenuous exercise, the distended abdomen does not seem to disappear for many people.

When I was in my twenties, I had a little potbelly. I had a nice figure, except for this protrusion. I started dating a weight lifter at this time, who developed a wheel with a handle on each side for me to use to flatten my abdomen.

I used it faithfully daily for three months.

My belly became as hard as a rock, but it still protruded! At that time, I had a bowel movement once every five days; this was the reason for my potbelly.

Now I am a senior citizen, yet I eliminate one to two times daily, and my belly is flat. I have had thousands of cleansings since 1971.

Internal cleansing as Clinical and Diagnostic Aid

Internal cleansing can be an aid in many clinical procedures, which now are only poorly facilitated by enemas.

In *The Nutrition and Dietary Consultant*, it is the professional opinion of Dr. Donald J. Mantell that colonics are one of the most important "treatment modalities" available for a multitude of health problems. He advocates colonics as a diagnostic tool to ascertain certain information about digestive and clinical disorders.

He states colonics cleanse the colon, making early detection of colorectal cancer easier. It does this by facilitating diagnostic procedures such as sigmoidoscopy, colonoscopy, and barium X-rays.

132

Testimonial

Rapid Recovery From Surgery

Recently, I underwent corrective surgery. Despite the severity and depth of the surgical cuts, my healing and my recovery were almost miraculous. The doctor, my family, and my friends were amazed that I was able to quickly return to work and my normal routine, without the trauma and pain the majority of surgical patients suffer. I attribute this to a clean, detoxified body

Signed
Teresa

Post-operative internal cleansing is especially important for patients who have general anesthesia. The bowel is usually traumatized and shuts down under a general anesthetic. In this state, it quickly becomes constipated.

Internal cleansing could help eliminate this serious problem. Likewise, lungs could clear out faster, preventing the potential for pneumonia.

The irony is that periodic internal cleansing and correct diet could possibly have prevented the vast majority of surgical cases.

The Healing Crisis/Cleansing Crisis

Many people go through a "healing crisis" or some call it a "cleansing crisis." This experience can be mild or intense. A healing crisis is inevitable; some experience it within hours of their first internal cleansing session, some later. It usually does not last longer than twenty-four hours.

The healing crisis happens because the body is finally releasing all the toxins and poisons it has been accumulating for years into the blood and kidneys.

During this time, a patient may experience one, or more of the following symptoms: fever, aches and pains, headaches (you may want to place a slice of lime against the area of the headache and many clients have stated this has

133

stopped the headache) joint pains, pimples, boils, light-headedness, lethargy (obviously, this is simulating the feeling of sickness and one does not feel like doing much), weakness, insomnia or sleepiness, flu or cold symptoms, runny nose, fever, chills, sweats, nausea, or excess gas. I always remind my client that these conditions are very temporary and symptoms can leave within 24 hours followed by a feeling of well-being and excess energy.

This is all brought on because the free radicals (those little molecular marauders that age you with oxidation) and various toxins are leaving the body. It is sometimes said that a client will feel worse before feeling better - but I know that my clients do feel better, especially afterward!

Perfect Health

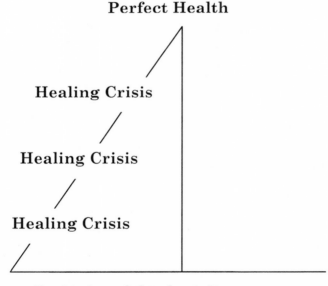

Healing Crisis

Healing Crisis

Healing Crisis

Beginning of the cleansing program

I present the complete list of healing crisis symptoms so my client will become aware of what is going on if the crisis occurs. Many people are never aware of experiencing a healing crisis. If

134

one does experience this event, I advise perseverance. This too - pardon the pun - will pass.

The healing crisis is brought on by two
things: the juice fast or modified diet and the actual physical stimulation of the internal cleansing. Most people experience similar sensations
while just fasting, which is why many people object initially to the fast.

The most difficult part of a fast seems to be
going without food - fighting the hunger pangs.
Some clients arm themselves with an herbal arsenal to keep hunger satisfactorily curbed. After 48
to 72 hours, the hunger subsides.

Some clients expect the healing crisis, even
want it. When it happens, they will know what it
signifies and they can cheer; thus, when all is said
and done, my clients will have taken a solid step
on the road to optimum health and anti-aging.

Testimonial

Suffering from Boils Gone

Dear Millan:
*I have suffered with boils on my butt for
three years. I have gone to my family doctor for
help but to no avail.*

*My family Doctor would give me penicillin
pills. The penicillin caused the boils to dry, but in
a few days they would return. The boils were very
painful. I had a hard time sitting, walking and
sleeping. I felt hot and sick daily.*

*I have had six internal cleansing sessions
from you and I am presently on your cleansing
program. Since I have been on your cleansing program, I have not had one boil. The pain I have suffered in my back for twenty-seven years has decreased. I feel tremendously relieved.*

*I am so grateful I am doing this cleansing
program. My life and health have really improved.*

Relaxing Bath

If a client does not experience the healing crisis right away, it just means it probably will take a little longer to detoxify, maybe two or three more cleansing sessions than the usual recommendation.

A couple of steps that can be part of detoxifying are relaxing Epsom salt baths and abdominal wraps. After the first day of fasting or modified diet, a warm bath is just the ticket to relax all that stress away. This bath will also begin to release toxins out of the body.

The following are general guidelines that I have suggested to my clients who want to enjoy the benefits of a soothing Epsom salt bath:

1. Fill the tub with comfortably warm water. It should be hot enough to last awhile, but not so hot that it is uncomfortable.
2. Empty a full box of Epsom salts into the water, distributing it evenly.
3. Climb in, stretch out and soak for an hour. This will open up all the skin's pores and eliminate toxins and poisons. Without even soaping, the effectiveness of this treatment can be seen in the dirty ring and dark water at the end of the bath time. All that junk was just excreted out of the body!
4. A quick, warm shower may be taken to rinse off any residue, which might clog pores again.
5. After bathing and before retiring, gather a bottle of castor oil, a roll of plastic wrap, and a heating pad.
6. Spread the castor oil on the abdomen. Wrap the plastic completely over the castor oil, then place the heating pad over

136

the wrapped abdomen and turn it on to gently heat for about one hour. Relax.

The combined action of the castor oil and the heat penetrates into the intestine and softens encrusted fecal matter, loosening it from within the convolutions and pockets of the colon. This helps loosen encrusted matter during the next internal cleansing sessions. Some of it may even be so well softened and loosened it will begin to come out during the next natural bowel movement.

Dr. Harvey Kellogg, founder of the Kellogg Cereal Company and Kellogg Sanitorium, in Battle Creek, Michigan, says in his book, *Colon Hygiene,* " that out of the twenty-two thousand operations he has personally performed, he has never seen one, single, normal colon.

Testimonial

Extended Healing Process

Dear Dr. LaBeau:
I write to you at this time to THANK YOU personally for your referral to Millan Chessman. I found Millan to be very supportive of my concerns and VERY knowledgeable about this cleansing procedure, but also very gentle and caring. She has extended my healing process through the internal cleansing services she provided.

Sincerely
Mark D.

Dr. John Christopher, a renowned herbalist, and author of *Three Day Cleansing Program* and *Mucusless Diet*, said he knew of a man who went on a cleansing program and noticed a certain type of berry coming out of his colon. After examination, the man positively identified it as one of the exotic berries he had eaten during the war on a South Sea Island twenty years earlier.

137

When my clients go through our cleansing program, they can expect to have a slightly full feeling. Taking place is softening of the bowel, which breaks away any old matter stashed in the pockets of the colon's walls.

Clients sometimes do not eliminate 2 days after a cleansing program.

CHAPTER TEN

Quote: Our knowledge of past history can determine our destiny of the future.
Millan Chessman

NUTRITION AND DIET GUIDELINES

Some clients, despite eating junk foods, continue to do internal cleansing, expecting it to be a "panacea" or cure-all. While there are undeniable improvements with every series of treatments, they are not as beneficial or obviously, as long lasting. I have one client who eats junk foods regularly, then comes in for internal cleansing.

The ultimate goal, the real reason for doing internal cleansing in the first place, is to cleanse and enable the body to assimilate more efficiently the nutrients it receives, leading to better health and longevity.

Internal cleansing is just an initial preparation for the complete program, real success, and final results. So, if individuals do not change their diet, internal cleansing only has a limited effect on their overall well-being.

As you read earlier, bad health is largely the direct result of a bad diet. Our standard American diet is a major reason so much ill health, unnecessary pain and suffering exist in this country. With the proper nutrition, America could be a country of radiant, vigorous, healthy people, many living well into their hundreds. I am aware that we live longer than we did in the 1800's, but please realize that with our extended years comes poor health, pain, and sickness. Who wants to live longer (and live longer sicker) under those conditions?

Simply put, our bad diet is due to a lack of whole, fresh foods - fruits, vegetables, nuts, seeds, legumes, and grains. Flesh foods, dairy products, refined sugar, processed, chemical and preservative-laced foods are the cause of our sluggish guts, our collective colon crisis, and the rise in cancer. In other words, if it says, "enriched," don't eat it.

Testimonial

Overweight and Constipated

My name is Myrna. I have been overweight and constipated since childhood.

When I was a teenager, I grew to two hundred pounds. I started taking amphetamines and other drugs for almost fifteen years to lose weight and keep it off. I then started suffering skin problems. Brown patches covered my body.

I found out about fasting, internal cleansing, and became a vegetarian.

With the combination of diet and internal cleansing, my skin cleared. I also suffered allergies, and because of the cleansing, they are gone.

Signed,
Myrna

Conditions such as: abdominal pain, especially on the right side, weight that just will not come off, a persistent pot belly, uncontrollable food cravings, overeating without feeling satisfied, bloatedness, excess gas, poor or increased appetite, coated tongue, unexplained recurrent nausea, pseudo-hypoglycemia, food sensitivities, asthma, chronic bronchitis or other respiratory problems such as chronic cold or flu-like symptoms, sinusitis, common headaches or migraines, hypersensitivity to light, smoke, or perfume, and allergies, can be benefitted by internal cleansing.

140

The Lean Lifestyle
For most of our history, until the last century, life was hard. It normally demanded great expenditures of sweaty and exhausting physical labor. This tended to keep workers too lean to sustain long life. Average life expectancy until the last century was only forty years.

Testimonial

Weight Loss Results

I have received a series of ten internal cleansing sessions and did the detox program. I have suffered from migraine headaches and obesity in the past. Now the migraines have incredibly diminished and I have lost twenty pounds. My out-of-control eating is behind me now.

Last week I saw a friend I had not seen in over a month, and she said, "What have you been doing? Your face looks glowing, and I can tell you lost weight." I did not want to tell her I've been getting internal cleansing, because I knew she wouldn't understand. She is not an open-minded person. I just told her, "I've changed my diet." I feel great now.

Valerie

In this century, lifestyles and diet have radically changed. Most of us in the Western world do not toil at backbreaking physical labor twelve hours a day. Most people in undeveloped countries still see Americans living the life of the unimaginably wealthy.

And we are fat to prove it!

This is because we eat flesh foods and dairy products in far greater proportion to plant foods.

Consequently, we are fat and dangerously unhealthy. The way to health for us in our society and its lifestyle is through plant foods and exercise.

141

Testimonial

Weight Loss and Allergy Relief

I could not believe allergy tests revealed I had forty allergies! That was two years ago. Last year I undertook a series of doctor recommended shots. Still, I continued to feel half-dead, weak, sick, and had no energy.

I had constant colds, a runny nose and sore throat.

When I began internal cleansing, lots of stringy old feces and ropy stuff came out. I followed my colon hydrotherapist's detoxification program to the "T." I have since lost ten pounds - a pleasant surprise - and people at work have commented on how good I look. They say that my eyes are brighter and my skin looks better.

Last night I saw an old beau who had not shown much interest in me previously. He appeared very interested, attentive, and commented on how well I looked!

Yesterday I went back to my doctor. He did the allergy tests again and discovered only two allergies! He said, "Whatever you're doing, keep doing it, because it's working!"

I must say the whole colon cleansing program has been beneficial. For once, my bowel movements are regular and elimination is easier. I am happier and life, overall, is more balanced.

I have always been a compulsive eater, and finally my appetite is more in control thanks to the cleansing. It is such an exhilarating feeling to have good health and energy.

Signed,
Christy R.

Shortcomings of Previous Diets

There are many weight-loss diets, and if you are like me and most of America, you have tried them all. Health officials are alarmed that after two decades of fad diets, exercise programs, fashion demands, and "fat-free" foods, Americans are still overweight. Moreover, people are making peace with the realities of human, physical bodies that were never intended to look like skin-draped skeletons.

In short, all those calorie counting diets are a pain and do not work.

Starvation and protein diets have failed totally. Ninety-five percent of those who lose weight gain it all back, plus more. It has been proven time and time again. Behavior modification, while proffering some good tips and recommendations, just does not meet the needs.

The isolation of radical diets is anathema to human social makeup; meals should be social, relaxing, and relationship-building affairs, shared for enjoyment. Towards that end, a healthy diet is worth the effort, and makes long life worth living. In other words, a healthy body makes life enjoyable.

Good health is attainable through internal cleansing, a healthful diet, and exercise. There is no calorie counting, starving, or sweating.

A clear head, a clean body inside and out, health, enjoyment, and longevity - through this program one can have it all. It may take clients a few weeks, but it does happen, and does people a lifetime of good.

The gradually restored health of the internal cleansing program seems to fly in the face of our "I want it NOW!" society and anyone looking for "instant" results will be disappointed. But it compares favorably to the disappointing process of losing ten or twenty pounds in a month, feeling great about it, and then, in horror, seeing all the weight and more climb right back on within two weeks.

My clients experience success with this program of internal cleansing, detoxification, cleansing herbs, and changed diet.

For the most part, the fruits and vegetables portion of the internal cleansing diet are handled on the client's own. Whenever possible, store-bought produce should be organically grown.

If more people demanded their grocers to stock organically grown produce, then bought it from them faithfully, more grocers would make the effort to get it and make it cheaper.

Remember, the bottom line is profit. If there is no profit in selling healthy foods, the grocer cannot be expected to stock them. The consumer must make the effort to make it profitable for the merchant.

The issue of which grains are best to eat and supplement the diet rages on; and most of us need guidance here. Certain fiber herbs can be used for bulk, if need be. Rice, oats, millet, barley, and brown rice are wonderful in this capacity.

Testimonial

Individual Difference

An instance comes to mind of a hospital administrator in her mid-forties. She heard about internal cleansing and decided to try it. She had a lot of problems - stress, lack of energy - and was continually upset. Following my instructions to a "T," she had a series of cleansing sessions and observed the recommended diet and cleansing program.

After a few sessions, this woman started to eliminate a lot of old fecal matter, shed weight, and her energy level improved. Her disposition changed. She was more optimistic, and a lot happier. By the time she had completed her series, she was a changed woman.

Interestingly enough, a month later her twenty-two-year-old daughter came in for a session (the two were living together). The daughter said, "You know, when my mother first came to you, she was impossible to live with. She would argue, and she was crabby. She was miserable. Now she is more pleasant to be around; she is easy to get

144

Potent Herbs

We need to remember that herbs form the basis of numerous refined pharmaceutical drugs. Some doctors marvel at the potency of herbs, and compare their few negative side effects to the processed and refined drugs prescribed, which often have many side effects. There was a time when orthodox medicine dismissed past discoveries like vitamin C, the benefits of doing aerobic exercise, and a high fiber diet. In addition, the contributions of Omega 3 and beta-carotene for combating cancer were scoffed at.

The Cleansing Herbs

Psyllium is a cleansing herb and should be used strictly when doing internal cleansing. I never recommend it as a regular fiber, but advocate its use only during this time to initially expand the colon and push old matter through. This expansion of the colon causes a slightly bloated feeling. I tell my clients this is good, and should be expected.

The psyllium forms a gel-like substance, expands the bowel slightly, and attaches onto the stool in pockets. Bentonite is then taken to detoxify the system through the alimentary canal. But psyllium taken at the recommended dosage for longer than seven days loses its effectiveness.

I have seen people time and again take prescribed doses of psyllium only to clog their colons - all because they do not follow up with colon cleansing.

I recommend wheat-grass tablets or good quality barley powder and flax seeds. These keep the bowel doing what it should, helping it along, and ensuring that nothing gets clogged in the colon.

Wheat grass tablets also contain every vitamin and mineral there is. Each pill contains eighteen of the twenty amino acids, which means it has more protein than beef. Moreover, it has twice the fiber of bran and a lot of chlorophyll. And, price for price, it cannot be beaten. Only barley powder compares.

The cleansing herbs my clients take, in conjunction with the overall colon cleansing program, help to remove excess mucus in the small intestine.

In some cleansing programs, my clients undergo one round of taking the cleansing herbs - five days on and five days off - while simultaneously having colon cleansing. This regimen really gets rid of all that old sewage.

Remember, a sluggish colon goes into renewed peristalsis with the internal cleansing program (internal cleansing in combination with the modified diet or juice fast and the cleansing herbs).

Testimonial

Migraines & Enlarged Liver Resolved

Dear Millan:

I came to you on doctor's orders with 2-3 migraines a day and a very enlarged liver due to two tumors. After I went to your clinic for 7 days and did the internal cleanses, my liver was normal size and I had renewed energy and a new outlook on life. The most dramatic event I experienced was that there were no more migraines. Do you know how free I feel to not constantly have migraine medication stashed in every vehicle, jacket, purse, and any available drawer in the event a migraine punches through? I do not even have a current pre-scription for my migraine medication. This is truly amazing!

Thank you for your patience, and knowledge. Promise you'll never stop having this service available to the general public! Thank you again!!!!!!!!!

Signed,
Detective Nanci L.

Dispelling a Myth about Meat-eaters

People have come to me for colon cleansing, and more than one person has told me vegetarians are much nicer and better people than meat-eaters.

Do not misunderstand; I am an advocate of a plant-base diet. I believe the body is designed for a vegetarian diet, but I know some meat-eaters who are the most loving people, with more kindness and consideration for others than themselves. They are active in standing up for the injustices of this world. They are out there caring for the down and out.

On the other hand, I have seen strict vegetarians who are only into themselves, who are deceitful, dishonest, and selfish.

I would trust them as far as I could throw them.

Many others have told me they are doing colon cleansing because their guru has told them this would make them better individuals. Better for whom? Themselves?

To me, a better person is one who will reach out and touch the lives of those who are suffering, who is volunteering to help the needy, to protect the child from molestation, to fight against the wrongs in the world – that is real love. People of love do this because they care and expect nothing in return.

I hear a lot about love. It is only a word, but love is action.

147

Psoriasis gone

Bob, my husband, had psoriasis all over his body for years. His father, brother, and sister all had bad cases of it. Bob had inherited a genetic propensity for psoriasis. We can inherit the weakness but we do not have to develop the actual disease! Bob wore long pants and long sleeves when we would go to the islands and played golf. He never went to a pool, never went to the beach. He had to wear these long clothes. It was horrible. And he lived with it because he believed the doctors who told him psoriasis was incurable. I went everywhere to try to find a cure. I could not believe nor accept anything less. I just could not.

We went to a nutritional doctor. He told Bob to eat stir-fry and take vitamins, and then he was going to get well. We believed him. But Bob's body was still covered with scabs.

For a year we searched. There were no answers. Then we went to the Holy Land, and when we came back, my husband looked like he had leprosy. I was so scared. I could not believe it. I said, "Let's pray before we do anything," and we did. This particular morning, we thought he was dying. I prayed that morning to God that something would happen. I just felt like Bob was dying and I was dying with him. I then remembered a woman I had met at a health lecture I gave on vitamins. She had gone to a doctor, and he got her off all the drugs she was taking. I heard her, but did not pay much attention because I was trying to present the lecture. So later, when I got back in the car, God began to speak to my heart. An audible voice literally screamed at me, "Call Dr. ____!" who was the doctor this lady had recommended. Bob and I discussed it and he decided to see the doctor. The doctor said, "Do you want to get well? Do internal cleansing." Internal cleansing was available at that office, so Bob began internal *cleansing, immediately. We had no idea what was in store. Bob came home and began the dietary cleansing program. As far as we were concerned, if this was not going to benefit him, he was dead. There was no other answer.*

Bob took one colon cleansing every day for six weeks and diligently ate nothing but raw vegetables, fruits, grains, nuts, beans, and legumes. He began to see the sores going away. At the end of six weeks, Bob had no psoriasis.

Signed,
Joanne

Bob's story, as told by his wife, reflects how internal cleansing helped him with psoriasis.

It has been over five years, now, and he does not have a sore on his body.

Sadly, not many people properly maintain this crucial internal chain reaction of nutritious food and health, and I can list at least two reasons why:

1. We need to educate ourselves, keep up with new research study results, learn the warning signs of bad health, and consult knowledgeable health practitioners in the area of preventive medicine. We should have appropriate tests run for diagnoses, and generally take active roles in the decisions of our own health.

   A first step should be to start with prevention. Grandma's old adage of "an ounce of prevention is worth a pound of cure" has no greater application than to our own health!

2. Most of us are unaware of the chain reaction - the cause and effect - of food and health. The human body is a wonderfully complex machine that over millennia has responded to changes in the environment.

   This human machine is remarkably durable, able to withstand abuses both from nature and self, but after many

149

years, insults to its integrity manifest finally in disease and disablement. The antidote is a nutritious diet and exercise.

While there is a latent period between what one eats and its eventual, cumulative effect on the body, without correction these effects will result in premature aging, disease, misery, and even premature death.

The health benefits of a changed diet are greater and more quickly felt, because with a good diet and internal cleansing, damaged tissues can begin to repair themselves. They may actually reverse aging and disease.

Testimonial

Testimonial from a Sufferer of PMS & Spastic Colon

Two weeks before my period, I would get irritable, with radical mood swings. I had pain and itching in the lower bowel area. Bloating caused weight gain and disoriented me.

I had an upper and lower GI and was given medications for my spastic colon condition. I was also treated for pre-menstrual syndrome. For three weeks now, I have had internal cleansings, and altered my diet. I had no pain before or during this menstrual period. I did not experience the bloating, disorientation, or mood swings. This is miraculous!

Anonymous

Evidence of our cultural proclivity for bad diet is all around us. It is a notorious fact that Americans are out of shape and lead the world in diseases such as cancer, heart attacks, and digestive disturbances. HEALTH AUTHORITIES NOW STATE 80% OF THE AMERICAN PEOPLE ARE OVERWEIGHT. These health disasters are virtually unheard of in "undeveloped" countries. Unfortunately, when any of these populations be-

150

come suddenly wealthy and begin to incorporate a Western diet into their lives, as well as a higher standard of living, these diseases begin to show up.

Obviously, something is terribly wrong with the food we eat. Yet, western medicine ineffectively continues to treat separate, isolated symptoms of individual diseases (by specialty, no less), and ignores the root dietary causes. Our medical institutions do not adequately understand the concept of prevention, especially prevention through better nutrition. This lack of knowledge is difficult to understand, especially given the clear results of extensive studies released over the past three decades directly linking disease to diet.

For this reason, some wholistic health practitioners suspect why the established medical profession stubbornly insists on the status quo: fewer health problems will naturally mean less call for the services of doctors and specialists. In turn, there would be a resulting loss of revenues, not only for physicians, hospitals, and their personnel, but pharmaceutical companies, as well.

The pharmaceutical industry is a $1.5 trillion industry, whereas vitamins and minerals make up only a $4 billion market. While standard markup on vitamins is forty percent, the pharmaceutical industry markup is eight-hundred percent!

Furthermore, powerful lobbyists for the dairy, meat, and sugar industries, as well as other large food manufacturing interests, promote huge advertising campaigns with limitless funds and government subsidies, not just here in the United States but all over the world. Our government even subsidizes advertising of alcoholic products, among other things, abroad.

Meanwhile, proponents of health, prevention and proper diet, struggle to make an impact in their local backyards. They do so without strong financial backing, and often with the disapproval

151

and harassment of both the medical establishment, media and the government.

So, for the time being, you will have to seek
good health on your own, without the help of na-
tional campaigns and in-your-face advertising.

Testimonial

From Suicide Tendencies to Health & Happiness

*Dear Millan: This letter comes with many special
thanks to you and yours. Thanks for what you did
for my friend Christina. It would be too much to
say the complete story about Christina. I will tell
you just a little. She was born with a damaged digestive system. Over the years, (she is now 48) her
digestive system was continuing to cause her more
problems, up to the time she was not able to defecate in a natural way. She felt she would not be
able to survive with her colon problems. She has
several big pockets on both sides of her colon and
her transverse colon was collapsed, pushing down
on the bladder and stopping it from working effectively. Thus, she does not urinate in a natural way.
She has a toxic liver and damage to her kidneys.*

*The last three years, I tried to help Christi-
na, to teach her to understand proper nutrition
and problems that she has developed. Her strong
will to live, the desire to overcome the sickness,
drove her finally to the U.S., as she didn't find
help in Germany.*
*In March, she bought her ticket to San Diego.
About two weeks before arriving, she was so
stressed, so afraid, so tired of living that she did
not want to come. She didn't want to be a heavy
burden on my husband Bob and me.   When she
arrived in San Diego, she had not been able to
empty her bowel for more than two weeks. She
didn't sleep, didn't eat, and didn't drink. She was*

152

so desperate that she didn't want to come, and in her mind she wanted to take her life, to commit suicide. Her husband and her brother convinced her to come to California. They did not know that she was thinking of suicide.

Christina had only 10 cleansing sessions. What a wonderful job you did. What a wonderful transition she made which is so visible. She has since gone back home.

She called me last week to say thank you again to all of you for the most wonderful thing that happened to her during the time of being in San Diego. She has more energy. She is more positive, is looking forward to getting better each day. She is happier and healthier. She sounds so optimistic and is truly grateful for the care you gave her.

Thank you for your love, your heart and friendliness. Thank you for the greatest job done on internal cleanse for my friend.

May the joy you gave Christina be given to you!
God bless
Signed, Wanda

Breaking with Traditional Diet

Admittedly, traditions and habits are hard to break; we become so used to particular foods of our families and culture. But the cheese and animal dishes of our youth could eventually cause heart attacks and hardening of the arteries; in addition, if we cling to bad toilet habits through prudery, it seems clear we are setting ourselves up for disease.

In the long run, it is easier, wiser, and kinder to our bodies and families to make wise choices for good change and health.

Capitalism and free enterprise, while the best, make it possible, even imperative, for food businesses to cater to the tastes of the ignorant consumer, rather than to products that support good health. Our culture consists of pleasure. The slogan, "If it feels good, do it," may not be articu-

153

lated as much as it was recently, but the philosophy certainly is fixed within our behavior. We take great pleasure in creature comforts, and in how things feel.

Food gives us great pleasure; it satisfies the taste buds and is socially acceptable, moral, and legal. It is maybe the one thing we like that is not immoral or illegal! But the wrong kinds of food are still wrong for our bodies and destroy our health. Taste is not everything.

Believe me, taste buds can adapt to healthy foods and really enjoy them. Just be patient. Persevere. With today's modern methods of processing, preserving, and packaging foods, food manufacturers can produce more food, ship it further, and store it longer than ever before. The food industry produces more newer foods than ever and in even greater quantities.

Most of this food supply is killing us slowly.

Testimonial

From Fat Food Cravings to Healthy Eating

Does the following anonymous case sound familiar?

Before I started internal cleansing I had incredible cravings for fat foods. I put on weight. My appetite was irregular, swinging to extremes. I was craving very specific foods, but eating gave me no satisfaction. The cravings continued.

When I started internal cleansing, everything changed. My eating satisfied me. My cravings changed and my desire to eat good, healthy food became more acute. Now, I eat only when I am truly hungry.

Anonymous

The makers of antacids have never had it so good; people today are leading more dangerously unhealthy, stressful lives. It is practically a no-win, lose-lose proposition for someone in today's society to try to adjust to a healthy diet. But it can be done! It just takes discipline, determination, and a desire to feel great.

Testimonial

A Former Varicose Vein Sufferer

Dear Millan,
I had suffered in the past with puffy varicose veins. They were ugly and embarrassing. I did your cleansing program of ten sessions.I am happy to report, and admittedly shocked to observe, these varicose veins are no longer puffy. Many are totally gone. Thank you!

Signed,
Mary

After Cleansing: A Gradual Change towards a Healthy Diet
So, where does one start on this proactive, healthful diet? First, of course, is that initial visit to the colon hydrotherapist to thoroughly, internally cleanse the body. Next, with her help and guidance, is to completely revamp the diet and lifestyle.

Any changes must start gradually after completion of the cleansing program.

Moderate exercise should be planned into the day; clients are not training for a triathlon, but they should at least walk, swim, or bicycle vigorously for twenty to thirty minutes, three to five days a week to get the heart pumping, lungs working, and blood circulating.

The most important aspect of lifestyle change must be the client's new diet. Clients find when they eat right, weight drops and cravings for the wrong foods disappear. Dr. Gordon Tesslor, in his book, *Lazy Person's Guide to Better Nutrition,* states the following:

155

We can successfully lose weight and keep it off by eating vegetables, fruits, grains, liquids, raw nuts and seeds, even dried fruit, but no roasted nuts and seeds

Weight will come off ever so gradually, but, if one perseveres, it will eventually come off. What a wonderful way to eat, not going hungry, and yet lose weight. Exercise should be a part of this weight loss program.

Foods to be included at every meal are fresh, preferably organically grown, raw fruits, vegetables, and fruit juices; grains (including brown rice, oats, millet, barley, corn, wheat, etc.); legumes (including lentils, all kinds of beans, black-eyed peas, split pea, garbanzos or chick peas, raw, unsalted nuts and seeds).

Roasted, salted nuts and seeds are not natural to the body, so they are not assimilated and broken down correctly. Consumption of these products results in more fat conversion.

The Immortal Cell: Carrel's Discovery

Dr. T. De La Torre, in *Man's Return to his Garden of Eden*, says the following:

In 1912, Dr. Alexis Carrel of the Rockefeller Institute took a piece of the living heart of a chicken and proceeded to experiment to see if it was possible to maintain its life apart from the chicken's body. The piece of chicken's heart is given a daily washing to remove its waste products and then is supplied with the required elements of nutrition, and it grows, it grows, it grows - it grows so fast that it is necessary to subdivide it, for it would become so large that it would become difficult to continue the experiment. This piece of chicken's heart was kept alive for over 26 years before the experiment was finally discontinued. During those 26 years the piece of a chicken's heart continued to grow with-

out giving signs of old age or loss of vitality, while many generations of chickens came into existence, lived their allotted time and returned to the dust whence they came. Moved by the marvelous discovery: 1. that if we supply the proper environment in the form of a daily washing out of the toxic waste products accumulating in the cells, 2. supply the proper nutrient media, it is possible to keep alive indefinitely a piece of chicken's heart, Dr. Carrel was inspired to formulate the Law of Perpetual Youth and Immortal Life in the following words: The Cell is immortal. It is merely the fluid in which it floats that degenerates. Renew this fluid at intervals, give the cells the required food to eat and, as far as we know, the pulsation of life may go on forever.

I cannot help but wonder if we could live forever without growing old, as Dr. Carrel and Dr. De La Torre believed and both indicated. Where are they today in 2011? These men were around in 1912 and Dr. De La Torre was obviously around in 1957, when his book was written. I wonder if they are still alive with the youthfulness they had then. Of course, we know this is impossible; nonetheless, this is something to think about.

Testimonial
Relief from Acute Arthritis Pain

Dear Millan:
I did your cleansing program with colonics for 7 days. Your treatments helped to relieve me from my acute arthritis pain. It is totally gone and I hope never to come back. Thank you, Millan.

Signed,
Vimla J

Thorough Chewing Aids Digestion

It is very important to chew food completely. It seems to be a problem here in this country. We are always in such a hurry with never enough time, so we gulp down our food and drink something to wash it down. This hinders the body from breaking down and assimilating nutrients in food and overworks the body.

Digestion begins in the mouth!
Earlier, I shared with you a story about a man, who lived into his hundreds and attributed his longevity to the slow and careful chewing of food. Does this mean if we chew our food slowly, we will live into our hundreds?

I honestly do not know. It could be!

Dr. Kellogg, in *Colon Hygiene*, says:

"Cows' milk is excellent for calves to which it is naturally adapted, but for many humans, it appears to behave almost as a poison. The probable cause is the very inability to digest the casein of cows' milk. Personal observation of numerous cases has convinced me that at least half of the people suffering from chronic disease cannot use cows' milk freely without serious injury.

One of the prominent symptoms arising from the use of cows' milk is a condition commonly known as biliousness. In this state, the tongue becomes coated, there is a bad taste in the mouth, the breath is foul, the bowel is inactive, and an examination of the stool shows considerable quantities of undigested casein undergoing putrefaction.

No doubt, extensive use of cows' milk, under the mistaken notion it is a valuable food for adults as well as for infants, actively increases constipation among civilized people. Putrefaction of undigested casein in the colon produces an alkaline condition, which paralyzes the bowel.

A nutritional consultant shared with me that if a calf is given homogenized, pasteurized milk from birth on, it would die before it reaches maturity.

What about the milk's additional fortified nutrients? Why would that not sustain a calf? If a calf were to die drinking store-bought milk, how can we expect our children to grow up healthy drinking the same?

Testimonial

Swollen Stomach Gone

Dear Millan:
I was in misery with my upper stomach totally swollen. I was very uncomfortable - feeling tired and constipated all of the time. I went to the M.D. and had all kinds of tests done and they couldn't find anything wrong. I finally went to the Gastroenterologist. Now after the internal cleansing sessions, changing my diet and taking cleansing herbs, I am amazed how much better my stomach feels. The swelling is completely gone. Before I couldn't bend over to wash myself because of so much pain on my side. Now there is no more pain and I can wash my feet and toes.

Lucy

My Experiences as a Breast-feeding Young Mother

When I was a young mother in the sixties, my baby was born during a time when breast-feeding was not accepted. Doctors told mothers to give their babies formula.

I was the outcast because I was the only one around nursing my baby.

Even though I knew little about the differences between the forms of feeding, deep within me I knew I was doing the right thing by breast-feeding my baby. I remember my in-laws thought I was disgusting, even though I was not exposing myself.

But my husband, mother, and father supported me. After all, my mother breastfed me!

One day, my neighbor asked if I could watch her baby for a short while. Since her three-month-old baby was the same age as mine, and I do love babies, I agreed.. Well, would you believe it, the moment that mother left, the baby started crying horribly.

I never let my babies cry, so this was very disturbing to me. I was beside myself as to what to do. I could tell that this baby was in extreme pain. It was colic (a condition of the digestive tract).

Finally, in desperation, I breast-fed the baby. She calmed down almost immediately, nursed for awhile, and then fell asleep. Not only was the breast milk nourishing for her, but also the warmth of my body was comforting to this baby.

Another incident at that time was with a friend who was a mother also. She told me her first baby suffered so much from drinking formula (cows' milk), that he was hospitalized for three months. How unfortunate.

Later, she was pregnant with her second baby. I pleaded with her to breast-feed the coming one, so it would not suffer like her first-born. She said she would discuss it with her doctor and see if he approved .He told her no, that breast-feeding was dirty, unsanitary, and only animals and primitives living in the wilds did such a thing.

I, being a young assertive mother, went and told him, "You are not a woman nor have you ever breast-fed a baby. I have! You have absolutely no right to tell any woman not to give her baby the most natural start in life as mother's milk!" How dare him!

He just looked at me and chuckled. He was probably amused that this twenty-one-year-old woman was telling him how to be a good doctor. I mean, after all, I had no education compared to his years of medical school.

My friend had her baby shortly thereafter; sadly, one month later, that poor infant reacted so violently to cows' formula she also ended up in the hospital.

While I am talking about my experiences as a young mother, I want to share also that I had my baby at home, totally natural. It was wonderful. As soon as my daughter was born, I breast-fed her, laid her in her bassinet, looked at my husband, and said, "Gee, I'm hungry!" I then got out of bed, went into the kitchen, popped popcorn, and made a cup of hot chocolate. The next morning I arose and washed the bedding. (I do not recommend home delivery with your first child).

Storage of Body Fat
There is little fat on the internal cleansing diet. What fat there is does not convert to body fat; it is broken down and burned, not stored in fat cells.

Back in the ice ages, when our ancestors foraged for food, humans developed a means of protecting themselves against hard times.

When pickings were good (spring and summer) and when tribes wandered to southern, warmer climates, people ate a lot at one time, and their bodies stored the excess fat to burn in lean times (late autumn and winter months).

Bodies lined with fat were warmer (being insulated against the cold naturally), needed less fuel to generate warmth and burn energy in activity, and were better able to ward off disease. For centuries - in fact, until the last century - chunkiness was a sign of robust good health, joviality and wealth, (since only the wealthy could afford all the luxurious food they wanted).

As in days of old, a little fat in the female body is still necessary for proper menstruation and childbearing. Tradition was that fat females were revered and their likenesses worshipped and emulated because they symbolized fertility.

161

CHAPTER ELEVEN

Quote: When evil enters your presence, only the power of God disperses its darkness. Millan Chessman

FOODS

Chemically Tainted Food Supply

Do you know we use more chemicals in our food than any other nation in the world? Even those chemicals that have been outlawed here are used by other countries to grow foods for export to the U.S. We import these tainted foods, and then ingest those chemicals as well.

The food we eat directly impacts our health. These foods determine how well our intestines and colon absorb nutrients and discard waste products. The types of foods in our digestive tract, and how well they move, determine the efficacy of all other body organs and tissues, which maintain radiantly good health.

Basic Food Groups vs. Meat and Dairy Industry

Two of the largest and most powerful industrial lobbies in the U.S. are the American Beef Association and the American Dairy Association. American school children for decades have been brainwashed into thinking the proper four food groups were dominated in importance by meat and dairy products.

It is a cultural badge here in "good ol' U.S.A." that Americans - particularly men - hate vegetables. For instance, former President Bush stated publicly he hated broccoli, and later had to mend fences with vegetable's industry representatives. Still, no White House or State dinner Bush attended ever had broccoli on the menu!

And until a decade ago, the executive diet badge of honor, the domestic indicator that you had arrived at a position of success, wealth, and power was to be able to afford an ample supply of steak and lobster.

Milk was the all-American drink of youth and vigor, and is still promoted as "good for everybody," while cheese is a highly desired component of the all-American hamburger - the poor man's steak.

It was only recently that the Food and Drug Administration attempted to change the order of the four food groups, to emphasize the importance of fruits, vegetables, grains and other plant-based foods. But the beef and dairy industries howled so hard and loud that the ranking of proportions for each of the food groups was compromised.

Still, it is progress, after nearly one hundred years of beef and dairy monopoly on the nation's nutritional psyche.

The point of all this is to illustrate how invested we are as Americans to a false, dangerous myth of what good nutrition is and what it means. And we are paying the tragic price, through the, ah, rear. Somehow, we must make a concerted public effort to change our diets for the better. Our lives are at stake!

Hormone Additives

Much of our food contains hormones. Have you ever seen a man with breasts? Because he has eaten so much meat, those hormones respond to his body. Hormones are being added to milk cows. Inevitably, if you do not get hormones in meat, you will get them in dairy. This is not natural.

164

Legumes

Another new diet ingredient that one may be regarding with a wary eye are beans. I recommend eating legumes (or beans), although some health practitioners do not. Growing up, we ate a lot of beans in my family. They are a great source of protein.

But you do not want all that gas, for which beans are famous, right? Well, beans do not have to equal gas if you prepare them correctly.

For gasless beans, I do not recommend cooking them straight from the package. This method can cause gas, bloating, and digestive problems. Beans have an excessive amount of phosphorous, which is an irritant of the nerves, especially if eaten in abundance.

Here is my recipe for gasless beans:

Sprout your legumes before you cook them, both for gaslessness and for better nutrition. For greater taste enjoyment and nutritional variety, select different kinds of dry beans and mix them together with a portion of uncooked garbanzo beans.

Fill a large jar 1/4 full with the mixed beans. Fill the jar to the top with distilled water. Let it sit overnight.

The next day, empty the water and rinse the beans. With the beans still in the jar, place it on its side.

Cover the mouth of the jar with a lightweight, porous material (I use a piece of clean, discarded pantyhose that I cut to size and hold in place with a rubber band).

Rinse the beans three times a day for three days.

Soon, they will begin to sprout. When you see the little green sprouts shooting out of the softened beans' skins, it is time to cook them! This process has changed the chemistry of the beans, eliminating the gas problem by making them easier to digest. And you only need to cook them for about an hour, not all day.

Sauté some chopped onions, Himalayan salt and garlic in virgin olive oil, add to the cooked beans with seasonings.

IT'S DELICIOUS!

Prepared this way, the beans will not give you gas. Enjoy!

Recent studies and research show that organic coffee is good for you. I drink a large cup in the morning. Yes I love my coffee and I am so glad to read the studies that show drinking organic filtered coffee has proven to benefit memory retention and memory clarity. Yea!!!

Many times people have said to me, "I have to have my cup of coffee in the morning because it causes me to have a bowel movement."

Let me tell you if you had a cup of hot water with lemon and raw honey in it, you would also go to the bathroom, for this drink would stimulate your bowels to move as well!

It is not coffee that stimulates bowels to move, it is the heat of the liquid that spurs the digestive system to start moving.

Ginger tea is a wonderful treat in the morning and is also good for the digestive system. Add a little honey and it will taste delicious. Simply grate a rounded tablespoon of fresh ginger and spoon a rounded teaspoon of raw honey into a large cup of boiling distilled water. Stir and then filter through a sieve. Drink and enjoy. What a way to start out the day!

Treat your body well, and it will serve you well. Again, as one centenarian said, "do everything in moderation."

Searching For Health Foods

Ironically, among modern supermarkets, stacked to the ceiling with hundreds of thousands of food offerings, only a few remote shelves stock "health foods."

Think about it. If only these foods warrant the label healthful, everything else is not.

"Healthful" foods are rare, even in the fresh produce department. Because of modern growing methods and constant tweaking of natural endowments in color, size, and taste, these "natural" foods have very little nutritional value left.

Fruits and vegetables have been altered to make them bigger, more colorful, and less prone to bruising or spoiling. Plus, they have been sprayed with chemical herbicides, pesticides, insecticides and topical preservatives.

Such unnatural changes in our food supply present unknown health hazards and rob foods of their God-given taste and nutrition, not to mention genetically engineered foods. We don't even know when we are eating them or not. The only time you know for sure is if you buy organic.

The bottom line is, as with everything else in our material-oriented culture, the motive is profit. Growers' concern over consumers' long-term health is minimal, as long as food sells at good prices. After all, everybody has to make a living, and we are living in the most advanced, and wealthiest country, right?

The fast-food niche is the greatest offender in this crass, capitalistic scrabble for profit. With today's technologies, people live in a state of constant hurriedness - time is money and many must eat on the run.

So, they end up eating foods less suitable for the human body's consumption than ever before in history. Worse, these foods are prepared in terribly unhealthy ways (deep fat frying is NOT healthy!).

Dairy Products
Some of my clients absolutely have to drink milk or consume dairy products. In these cases, science dictates that they drink raw milk or eat raw butter or raw cottage cheese. Today, these products are carefully certified by the dairies. Raw milk has been consumed for thousands of years. The body can break raw elements down and assimilate the natural nutrients far more effectively than it can homogenized, pasteurized, and fortified milk.

Pasteurization kills the natural bacteria, which help the body digest these products. I question the nutritional benefits of such refined foods. The French do not use pasteurization, and they have very few problems with colon cancer or heart disease, despite a daily diet of dairy products.

Remember, flesh foods, processed food, refined sugars, and processed milk are mucus forming. Undoubtedly, bacteria thrive on excess mucus.

Animal Protein
A recent study on animal protein resulted in the following: *The arteries get clogged because of animal proteins in humans, and when that happens, blood flow is hindered. This includes the blood flow to the reproductive organs. In men, the results are not only low libido, but erections that are temporary or nil.*

A Diet for Internal Cleansing
I recommend to my clients a plant-based diet. It is the best plan for my clients' health. You may even find after a time on the plant foods that your body and your taste buds will actually reject the taste of flesh foods, eggs, milk, and cheese.

People do not realize they are actually addicted to flesh foods. That is why it is very difficult to stop eating it, and why they justify eating it. If you went without eating animal for any length of time and then went and ate it, you could become violently ill in your stomach, with excruciating pain. You may actually gag. It has happened.

Ignorance and misinformation are the true causes of ill health.

You may find well-meaning, but ignorant, folks blanch with concern and earnestly warn you that without animal sources of protein and calcium, you will harm your body.

But that is not so. Eating fruits, vegetables, grains, legumes, and raw seeds and nuts, will give all the protein and calcium the body needs, and in complete superior form.

Most foods in the diet for internal cleansing are composed of complex carbohydrates. Complex carbohydrates are high-fiber, low-calorie, and provide bulk in the digestive tract. These foods are very filling; therefore, on this diet, hunger is satisfied more quickly and completely.

Another advantage is these foods do not stay long in the digestive tract because of their high content of fiber. This roughage benefits the colon by "sweeping out with it" toxins and poisons.

And, as an added plus, fiber absorbs calories! Overweight people will see a beneficial weight loss once they change to a plant base diet.

Dr. Paavo Ariola explains in his book, *Are You Confused,* that a study was done on the performance of athletes and the effects of protein. The study showed that their performance improved after they switched from a 100-gram a day animal protein diet, to a 50-gram a day vegetable protein diet.

Japanese researcher, Dr. Kuratsune, found that 20-30 grams of protein in the diet per day is sufficient to sustain good health.

So what can too much animal protein do to your body?

Foul body odor, toxicity in the body, interference with the release of serotonin, it steals calcium, can cause intestinal putrefaction, vitamin B6 deficiency, arteriosclerosis, heart disease, kidney damage, arthritis, and low-libido in male and females.

The Max Plank Institute in Germany showed that many vegetables, fruits, seeds, nuts, and grains are excellent sources of complete proteins. Other research studies corroborate with this.

Soy beans, sunflower seeds, sesame seeds, almonds, potatoes, most fruits, and green vegetables contain complete protein.

It's important to remember these two facts:
1. Vegetable proteins are higher in biological value than animal proteins. For example, proteins in potatoes are biologically superior to proteins in meat, eggs or milk.
2. Raw proteins have higher biological value than cooked proteins. You need only half the amount of proteins, if you eat raw vegetable proteins instead of cooked animal proteins.

Soy

There seems to be a question of whether to eat soy as a substitute for animal protein; some say that it's not good to eat; however, I eat all kinds of soy products almost daily and am so grateful for the different kinds of foods it mimics. It has never harmed me or others that I know who use soy products. Remember, the Asians have had soy in their diets for thousands of years and are some of the healthiest people in the world.

A Vegetarian Times article states, "Soy is a genuine miracle food. In addition to its vast and varied culinary uses, recent studies show that certain compounds called isoflavones – which are found exclusively in soy – can lower cholesterol levels, relieve symptoms of menopause, prevent osteoporosis and fend off some forms of cancer. Soy is low in saturated fat and high in protein, as well as packed with important minerals like calcium and iron." It is important to make sure the soy you consume is organic. Eighty percent of soy grown in the USA is genetically modified.

I eat a lot of soy products. I absolutely love it. They don't get any healthier than me! I figure if it's good enough for the Japanese, it's good enough for me. They have been eating soy for more than five thousand years. This is something to think about. Remember they are one of the longest living races in the world.

170

Rotting Meat

Take a piece of meat, chicken, fish, any kind, and put it on your kitchen counter. Leave it there for a few days and see what happens. The stench will become unbearable.

Remember, if you were to eat that animal, it would likewise sit in your colon for days - sometimes even years - doing its job of rotting and stinking in your body.

Have you ever smelled someone's bad breath and caught the odor of feces? Do not think that because meat is properly refrigerated, the bad bacteria problem is resolved. Your warm body temperature creates a great atmosphere for destructive bacteria, which is in the flesh food.

Medical experts worldwide recognize the extensive degeneration of the body's absorption of putrefactive bacteria in the intestinal tract. Constipation, diarrhea, headaches, and other illnesses result from this problem.

Being symptom-free does not equal being toxin-free.

Not only can internal cleansing assist in restoring the physical body, research shows that eating too much animal interferes with the release of serotonin, which is what the brain needs to help with mental balance. If you or someone you know suffers from depression, mood swings, anxiety, stress, or insomnia – it's possible that a cleansing program will enable one to deal with the difficulties life doles out with the greatest of ease.

Vegetarians

A significant difference between a flesh-food diet and a vegetarian diet is that the latter is non-putrefying and not odoriferous. However, clients have come to me saying they are vegetarians but still have numerous problems.

Upon questioning them further, I discovered they drank tons of milk and consumed many fatty foods such as cheese, donuts, candy, french fries, sodas, and who knows what else. But "they are

171

vegetarians and proud of it." This does not make sense.

They might as well be septic tanks.

Those eating strictly vegetables, fruits, grains, legumes, raw nuts, and seeds have a diet that is non-putrefying. Fermentation takes place and forms harmless acids, which aid in proper bowel elimination. Typically, stools will have a slightly sour, non-offensive odor.

Nutritious food, preferably organically grown, fuels your body. But this fuel has to be converted from large, more or less hard and dry pieces into something small - on the molecular level - soft and moist before your body can use it.

Be careful about eating a lot of bananas. I once instructed a client to eat only fruits and vegetables two days before his internal cleansing session. This man went and ate bananas all day long. He became quite bound up because of all of the bananas he ate. He was really in a dilemma.

The body performs a process of transformation using a combination of chemical and mechanical (muscular) actions to break down food. This process begins the moment you put food into your mouth, although your body usually prepares for digestion before this happens. Remember, the colon is a muscular organ.

The lesson is that certain natural foods - bananas and cooked potatoes - are not easy to digest. For instance, a client should not eat potatoes thinking it is only a vegetable and nothing else; after all, their hydrotherapist told them to eat fruit and vegetables before internal cleansing, so why not? These starches slow down the cleansing effect on the body.

Taking Control of Our Bodies
It is terribly sad that we are conditioned in this country not to explore alternative health measures. Too often, a grim diagnosis causes us to give up, rather than pursuing the healing available to us from non-conventional sources.

172

For instance, fifty percent of Americans will be diagnosed with cancer. Cancer causes one death in the United States every 50 seconds.

Regarding another disease, the book *2001 Fascinating Facts*, reports:

As of 1977, diabetes was the third leading cause of death by disease in the United States. It has increased 50 percent since 1965, and today affects at least 10 million Americans. Of the 32 million Americans admitted to hospitals each year, some 1.5 million develop some disease that comes simply from being in the hospital. More than 15,000 people die of such a disease each year. So prevalent is a syndrome that doctors have given it a name - nosocomial disease, from the Greek word nosconium, meaning "hospital."

But there is a wide body of evidence to suggest that these diseases can be combated by internal cleansing and diet!

CHAPTER TWELVE

Quote: Be disciplined with yourself and patient with others. Millan Chessman

HOW YOUR BODY DIGESTS FOOD

Gary Lewkovich, D.C., tells of the experience of one of his patients whose constipation had advanced to a painful and debilitating stage:

We needed to clean out the severely impacted right side of her colon. In order to do so, it was imperative to get her on colon [hydrotherapy] right away.

For years, the patient had experienced abdominal pain, mood swings, indigestion, and an irritated ileocecal valve. Soon into the [cleansing] program, she no longer had pain in the abdomen, her moods stabilized, and she was digesting properly.

A post X-ray showed that, sure enough, the valve had closed.

Initially we advised avoidance of certain foods. Because her ileocecal valve was so irritated, we could not start right away to increase her roughage intake. We had to get the valve closed first and then work on increasing the fiber in her diet.

After the ileocecal healed and began functioning properly, the patient's diet included greater amounts of fruits and vegetables to keep it healthy. These foods keep digesting as they move along to the large intestine.

175

Digestion

When you think about, see, or smell foods you like, especially if you are hungry, your mouth begins to water. This is saliva, a clear, tasteless liquid that resembles water but is actually a chemical produced by the salivary glands in your mouth. Saliva carries a digestive enzyme that breaks down starches into simple sugar and begins to digest your food.

Saliva mixes into the food you chew. The food is reduced to a soft, moist, bland little ball which, when it is ready to be swallowed, is tossed to the back of your mouth where a reflexive muscle forces the food into your esophagus, beginning the downward muscular propulsion we call "swallowing."

The large intestine has three parts: the ascending, transverse, and descending. The cecum, which rises sharply on the right side of the abdomen, is the beginning of the ascending colon. The large intestine becomes the transverse colon as it crosses over at the liver to the left side of the abdomen below the stomach. It becomes the descending colon as it plunges about six inches downward on the left side to where the sigmoid is (usually as far as an enema can get). The intestine forms a loop called the sigmoid flexure, which opens into the rectum.

The rectum ends in the anal canal, just above the anus, the opening to the outside of the body. The anus is normally closed tightly by two contracted sphincters. When you need to pass the waste products from a meal, you consciously relax the anal sphincters, allowing elimination of the feces.

By the time the chyme (partially digested food) reaches the cecum, your body tries to glean every usable molecule of fuel it can. So, instead of simply shooting through the colon, the chyme, becoming feces (or part waste material) makes a tortured trip through a succession of pouches.

176

Actual digestion is minimal in the colon. Because of harmful bacteria activity on the waste material, feces remaining here too long begins to poison the body. These kind of feces are usually not waste products from fruits, vegetables, grains, raw nuts, seeds, or legumes.

Compared to the muscular activity of the previous parts of the digestive tract, the colon is less vigorous. But two or three times a day, if one is eating a healthy, high-fiber diet, a strong motion called a mass peristalsis is generally experienced, stimulated by the pressure of the fecal masses on the lower rectum, which first becomes distended with its load and then contracts against it.

The first of these peristalses is typically not noticed, but each succeeding mass peristaltic wave grows stronger until the need to use the toilet to relieve pressure becomes urgent.

Some people ignore or suppress these urges. Even if such a person eats a very healthful diet, this retention "discourages" the colon, which then tolerates the fecal mass and produces fewer and weaker peristalses. Suppression, may actually stop peristalsis altogether. If this happens, a person becomes constipated.

Lymph System
Another vital body system affected directly by digestion is the lymph system. It has its own circulatory system and performs some of the same functions the blood does, like carrying away waste products from cells.

Nutrition counselor and author of *The Colon Health Handbook*, Robert Gray, believes that the colon is the principal organ into which the lymph deposits its wastes. Gray further theorizes that the colon has a special ability to detoxify lymph.

This cannot be accomplished, obviously, if there is an accumulation of putrefying fecal matter in the colon. So, like the colon, the lymphatic system can contain stagnant waste material.

177

If you clog the colon - a detoxifier and portal for lymph - you also clog the lymph system, and the toxins are redistributed throughout the body, contributing to its poisoning.

Lymphatic Massage

My daughter Roxanne shares from experience:

When a client is given a lymphatic massage before internal cleansing, the lymphatic system releases a great amount of tiny mucus particles or a cloudy substance. This can be seen through the viewing tube.

Different substances always drain from the body after a pre-treatment of lymphatic massage.

My sauna clients dump a great amount of matter from the liver. Clients have gone to other colon hydrotherapists, receiving as many as fifty sessions. Neither cleansing herbs nor any cleansing program was ever recommended with their sessions.

I put one woman, with fifty prior sessions, on a cleansing program, and in four sessions she dumped a large quantity of waste the full forty-five minutes of each colonic. She said in all the other sessions combined she had not released so much as she had with my cleansing program.

As my daughter shared this story, I thought -- here is a client who had gone to a colon hydrotherapist with twelve years' experience yet still did not put clients on any kind of cleansing program to help rid the body of old fecal matter. How unfortunate to have a colon hydrotherapist who knows nothing about cleansing herbs or a good cleansing program!

Sweet Breath & Tummy Flat

A letter from a client's wife states:

> *My husband was a heavy meat and sweets eater who ate his biggest meal late at night. When he would come home from work, his breath smelled as if something had crawled into his body and died.*
>
> *It was awful! He also had a potbelly but was thin everywhere else.*
>
> *He did a nine-day juice fast monitored by Millan, herbal colon cleansers and colon hydrotherapy each day. She put him on a nutritious diet after his cleanse.*
>
> *Now his breath is sweet smelling, no matter what time of the day, even in the morning when he awakes. His abdomen is now totally flat*

Anonymous

In a healthy individual, the total time for digestion from mouth to anus, varies four to twenty-six hours, depending on what is eaten. Ideally, one should expect to have two to three bowel movements a day, usually after each meal.

Gas

Sometimes little bubbles furiously race by through the viewing tube of the colonic equipment. This is excess gas. Isn't it nice this is a closed system? During many sessions, clients note these gas bubbles. While it is natural to have a certain amount of gas, excess gas is not normal and is an indication of a toxic, impacted colon. Most excess gas is caused by fecal material in the colon, decomposing just like a carcass out in a field.

This offensive gas can be a byproduct of putrefied bacteria. These organisms break down and re-digest previously digested waste material that should have been excreted long ago. Stress, excitement, and anxiety can also cause excess gas.

Excess gas is a common experience of clients, and is something to be expected while on a cleansing program.

Certain foods like broccoli, cauliflower, onions, garlic, cabbage, and cucumbers can also cause gas. On the other hand, foods eaten in wrong combination can produce flatulence. Another possible cause might be a lactobacillus and coliform bacteria imbalance.

For all these reasons, it is normal to have some gas while on a cleansing program. Just hang in there—it is only temporary. When this period is over and the diet is changed, the stools and gas will no longer have an offensive odor.

The Problem of Gas

Many factors contribute to the problem of gas but according to Dr. Gary Lewkovich, "Gas is most often a sign of one or more flaws in the complex process of digestion, absorption or elimination." He suggests the following to reduce occurrence of gas:

1. *Do NOT eat quickly. Avoid stress while eating.*
2. *Chew your food thoroughly before swallowing.*
3. *Do NOT overeat.*
4. *Do NOT eat within two hours of bedtime.*
5. *Do NOT drink more than eight ounces of liquid with a meal.*
6. *Drink at least eight to ten glasses of pure water each day.*
7. *Eat your vegetables lightly steamed.*
8. *Avoid swallowing air as you chew or drink.*
9. *Avoid those foods that you have difficulty digesting.*
10. *Minimize sweets (cookies, candies, syrups, etc.).*
11. *Minimize fatty or fried foods.*

12. *Minimize alcohol and carbonated beverages.*
13. *Keep your meals simple, but vary them from day to day.*
14. *When using nutritional supplements, try to use the capsule or powder form, in preference to pills or tablets.*
15. **Exercise daily, but wait at least one hour after your meals to do so.*
16. **Eat when hungry, not according to the clock.*
17. **Use acidophilus - when indicated – to restore friendly colon bacteria.*
18. **Use digestive enzymes - when indicated - to help digestion of protein, fats and carbohydrates.*
19. **Use hydrochloric acid supplements - when indicated - to aid the digestion of proteins. Do NOT use it if you have an ulcer.*
20. **Keep your colon clean and healthy. Eat adequate amounts of appropriate high fiber foods but avoid laxatives.*

*Please consult with a Health Professional before using any suggestion with an *.

Testimonial

Gas & Bloating Gone

Dear Millan:
   A million thanks for your counseling and advice in regaining my health. For the last two years, I have been miserable with declining vitality and continuously uncomfortable with gas and bloating. In my desperation, I saw a Gastroenterologist at the rate of $l50.00 per visit. He actually gave me an injection directly into my abdomen to relax the clenched muscles and a couple of rather expensive prescriptions.
   In contrast, after the very first colonic my

181

stomach muscles relaxed. After only half of the detox/colonic series, I am experiencing a marked improvement in energy and sense of well being, not to mention a progressively trimmer waistline. I would think people would do this simply for the vanity of looking younger. This is a welcome lifestyle change, no longer craving junk food and empty nutrition snacks to truly enjoying wholesome food. I have the utmost respect for your profession and feel blessed in knowing you all. Thanks again and may God bless your important work!

Ron G

Digestion in Herbivores/Carnivores

Human beings need plant matter in their diet. If we compare the digestive tracts of herbivores to carnivores, we find that plant-eating animals tend to have rather long intestinal tracts, whereas flesh-eating animals have relatively short ones.

A carnivore's (meat-eating animal) short digestive tract suggests it was designed to reduce the time meat spends going through it. Logically, this also reduces the degree of putrefaction of fleshy waste products attained before elimination. Plant materials are easily digestible, so plant eaters have elaborate digestive systems to glean all possible nutrients from their diet.

Our human digestive tracts resemble those of herbivores - plant-eating animals - (this gives a possible clue as to why people who eat a lot of vegetables and fruits, grains, legumes, and raw nuts and seeds have fewer bowel and health problems).

A vegetarian's food does not tend to putrefy. However, meat rots in the digestive tract, spending more time going from mouth to anus, and, consequently, there are far greater opportunities for poisonous wastes to be introduced, absorbed and circulated in the bloodstream.

Weight Loss and Knowledge Acquired

My experience this last week with Millan's internal cleansing program has been transforming. Not only that, I feel great. I lost 8 lbs, and have learned about health from her. Her sensitive and caring spirit was uplifting. This was difficult at times because of my own beliefs of the so-called animal diet and how it affects my health. Millan walks the talk. She even fasted with my husband and me together.

I am blessed to have this experience with Millan and I recommend her services.

Thank You,
Aileen T.

Parts of the Digestive System

The digestive system consists of the alimentary canal and accessory organs. The colon is a part of the alimentary canal, which has an oral cavity, pharynx, esophagus, stomach, small intestine, duodenum, jejunum, gall bladder and cystic duct, common bile duct, pancreas, and spleen.

The colon has two functions: to absorb water, sodium, and other minerals for the body's electrolyte supply, and to receive and reduce the chyme from the small intestine and store it for subsequent discharge.

Abdominal Pain Disappears

In November, I was experiencing abdominal pain every day. It was very difficult to work or sleep at night.

After a month of pain, I decided to go to the

doctor. He put me on a lactose-free diet. I tried that for a couple of weeks, but that did not help at all.

After running further tests, my doctor still could not find anything wrong with me.

I experienced the pains throughout Christmas. I could not eat because the pain was so bad.

The last day of the year, I went to get colon hydrotherapy. I did not notice much difference at first, but one morning soon after, when I woke up, the pains had disappeared and they never returned after that.

Signed Paul

Elimination

The brain senses the rectum's distension and gives one the urge to have a bowel movement. Voluntary nerve impulses can inhibit the evacuation reflex, but this is a poor practice. Since the defecation reflex is weak, many voluntary muscles are called upon to assist the involuntary ones.

Constipation test

A charcoal test may be taken to determine the degree of constipation.

If the bowels move at 8:00 a.m., charcoal (purchased at any health food store) is taken then and again at 4:00 p.m. the same day. If some of the charcoal is not passed by the second morning, a person is regarded as constipated. The major portion of any one meal's residue should be expelled within forty-eight hours. Undue delay is failure to expel within a period of seventy-two hours.

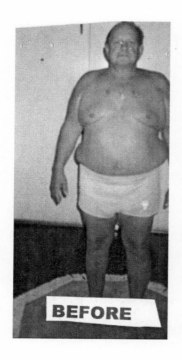 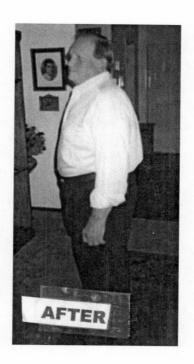

This client's appearance dramatically improved after internal cleansing.

Testimonial

A Client's Quick Relief From Bloat & Pain

First, let me thank you for the quick relief you gave me in my time of need. As you know, I was backed up and did not have a bowel movement for a week. This was causing me sharp pain day and night. Every hour, I was walking the floor with pains in my abdomen.

I felt so bloated that I did not want to eat anymore. Not being able to have a bowel movement is very serious. Something had to be done about it. My doctor recommended that I see you for several colon cleansing sessions. After the first session, I was able to sleep six hours straight without waking up. After the next few sessions, my bowel hab-

*its returned to normal! I can eat and sleep again,
thanks to internal cleansing!*

Signed,
Robert

Internal cleansing and Intestinal Mucus

Removal of mucus is not an initial objective in internal cleansing. The colon walls normally secrete the substance, and during the session the mucus secretion increases as the contractions of the colon cause the mucus-secreting goblet cells to release mucus.

After healing or toxin removal the thickened mucus can be sloughed off. Normal mucus coatings are not removed during sessions.

Colon X-rays

One X-ray showed piles of calcium tablets lodged in a patient's ileocecal valve. The supplements were a total waste of time and money because there was no benefit, only irritation.

X-rays show how twisted, looped, and ballooned the colon looks. After a series of internal cleansing, another X-ray will reveal the amazing difference in the shape of the colon. It will look more normal than before.

Colonoscopies are more frequently recommended and administered today to detect bowel disorders.

One M.D. who was a client of mine told me he participated in a bowel surgery where the patient had a huge blockage of waste. They removed a portion of her colon where the blockage was. To me that is barbaric! I believe internal cleansing would have removed the excess waste to resolve the problem.

Skin Brushing

It is very important to brush the skin while cleansing the body. A good skin brush can be bought at the health food store.

Because skin is the largest eliminator of toxins and poisons, you can be sure it is excreting a lot of these impurities. The only area to avoid brushing is the delicate skin of the face. There are special brushes available for this.

Testimonial

Acne sufferer benefited

Dear Millan,

It is just amazing to me to see that such a simple thing as internal cleansing, cleansing herbs, the special diet, and the skin brushing has improved the condition of acne I have suffered with. I have been to many dermatologists and they gave me different prescriptions, but nothing has made such a difference as your cleansing program. I do not feel embarrassed to look at people in the face with my new face.

Signed,
Hank

My clients skin brush daily on dry skin before bathing. All of the body, even the bottom of the feet, is brushed. With this daily routine, body skin feels refreshed and facial skin looks smoother and more radiant.

When I have a client with bad acne or pimples, I have found the greatest improvement on this condition is to daily skin brush all of the body, while cleansing.

When the body is detoxifying, the skin is working to eliminate. Skin brushing expedites the cleanse.

Testimonial

No More Skin Rashes

Dear Millan
    I have suffered from skin rashes forever. I then did a 7 day cleanse with juice fasting. The final results were that my skin rashes were gone. Both my husband and I lost several inches around our middle. As an added bonus, we felt as if we were on vacation while doing the entire cleanse. We want to thank you so much for your book.

Sincerely,
Gloria Carroll

CHAPTER THIRTEEN

Quote: Compassion is a sympathetic awareness of another's distress together with a desire to alleviate it. Millan Chessman

FRIENDLY FLORA

Economics of Internal Cleansing
Internal cleansing sessions take thirty-five minutes to one hour. Taking a laxative requires only a few seconds. Time is money. The benefits of colon hydrotherapy and its detoxification outweigh the time it takes to complete the sessions. As my father used to teach me, "anything worthwhile requires time and effort."

MIND GUT CONNECTION: WHY INTESTINAL BACTERIA MAY HAVE IMPORTANT EFFECTS ON YOUR BRAIN. (Friendly Flora)
There is a growing body of scientific evidence that early exposure to diverse microorganisms result in healthier immune systems. A new study may indicate that intestinal bacteria could have significant effect on the brain. So when you say you "have that gut feeling," you may not be too far from the truth.

A study published in the March issue of Neurogastroenterology & Motility examined germ-free mice—i.e. mice deprived of contact with bacteria at a formative age. The researchers observed changes in brain activity based on varying microbe levels. They also found germ free mice more likely to engage in risky behavior than mice with normal levels of intestinal flora. This bacteria may be influencing the behavior of these mice. Anybody who has ever listened to their gut when making important decisions, might be satisfied to learn of this biochemical evidence for the mind/belly connection. The vagus nerve that connects the brain to parts of the digestive system may be the conduit. This vagus nerve tells your brain how hungry you are based on what it senses in your belly. Could there be a connection to intestinal flora and depression? Further studies may show that to be the case.

Beneficial Implant (Friendly Flora)
With the prescription of an M.D. the procedure of a healthful implant is important.

The benefits of an implant of friendly flora which must be prescribed by a physician, includes the following: it balances the bacteria in the colon, sweetens the breath and rids the body of foul odors, creates digestive enzymes, effectively breaks down carbohydrates, controls candida, reduces bowel irritation, improves digestion and assimilation, manufactures abundant nutrients, reduces fermentation, maintains alkalinity and the necessary acidic condition of the colon, eliminates gas problems, raises the immune system, aids in production of lactose, and eliminates rashes from food. Flora Source, a manufacturer of friendly bacteria, states the following:

Mounting research continues to prove that the health and efficiency of the digestive system, and the immune system, depend on the complex interaction of "friendly" bacteria and balance in gastrointestinal ecology. Interaction of certain beneficial strains of bacterial cultures can aid in:

1. *Maintaining balance during and after the use of antibiotics, chemotherapy, sulfa drugs, and other harsh medication.*
2. *Relief and prevention of food sensitivities (including lactose intolerance),constipation, diarrhea, abdominal pain, bloating, gas, and digestive disorders.*
3. *Support for sufferers of candidia, Crohn's disease, and colitis.*

190

4. Production of enzymes and B-vitamins, and synthesis of essential nutrients, including vitamin K.
5. Calcium assimilation and hormonal balance.
6. Production of short chain fatty acids, supplying 5% to 10% of energy needs.
7. Control of enteric infections.
8. Re-establishment and maintenance of healthy vaginal flora.
9. Beneficial effects on cholesterol.
10. Stimulation of the immune system.
11. Digestive support while traveling.

Whey can also be implanted, which provides an environment enabling the friendly bacteria to multiply. Other beneficial ingredients can be implanted as well.

Remember, these medically prescribed implants get absorbed through the walls of the colon and ultimately into the bloodstream. In order to do its job, the implant should sit in the colon for at least ten minutes without eliminating.

Leslie Williams, former President of I-ACT, told me a study was done regarding internal cleansing. Ten participants, who qualified, participated.

Stool samples were taken to determine friendly flora content. As expected, many had none or very little. They received nine internal cleansing sessions each for one month. During that time, they were not allowed to take lactobacillus acidophilus or yogurt. After the 30 days, they took another stool sample. What they discovered was that their bacteria balance improved dramatically. The number one benefit they discovered was the hydration improvement, allowing the mucus to flow more freely in the body. This is a very impressive discovery and highlights some of the benefits of internal cleansing.

191

Friendly Flora and Putrefactive Bacteria

Toxins are eliminated by the stomach, the blood, the gall bladder, the small intestine, and other organs. The poisons combine with undigested food, thus passing through the body and into the large intestine.

The colon is the toxic dumping ground of the body. If pockets of the colon are impacted with excess sewage - stagnating for who knows how long - how can proper elimination take place? The body autointoxicates and it becomes a vicious cycle.

The body reabsorbs putrefying bacteria and cannot expel it. Have you ever smelled someone's dirty hair or reeking feet?

Invariably, these poor folks have a putrid BM bound up in their large intestine. Their stools likely result from a mixed diet of flesh foods, processed foods, refined white sugar, white flour and dairy products, and weigh about five ounces. In contrast, stools from the diet consisting of vegetables, fruits, grains, legumes, raw nuts, and seeds are double in weight, which is the fiber.

By the way, the healthy foods I have listed in this book are all fibrous foods, which absorb calories. A high-fiber, natural diet is like a broom sweeping your body clean.

There are more than one hundred and fifty different species of bacteria, which have been found in fecal matter. Of these species, more than a third posses pathogenic elements.

Colon hydrotherapists can implant lactobacillus acidophilus and bifidus cultures, at the end of each session, with the prescription of a physician. This restores and promotes the recolonization of G.I. flora.

Bacteria naturally dwell in your colon: the "friendly" group (mainly lactobacillus acidophilus, bifidus), and the preferably much smaller colony of anaerobic bacteria (E. coli II). Malabsorption and illness can result from an imbalance or absence of these bacteria. The ideal ratio should be four to one - lactobacillus acidophilus to E. coli II. Unfortunately, the typical American diet reverses that balance, resulting in health problems. When doctors prescribe antibiotics, friendly bacteria are destroyed along with the harmful organisms, yet most M.D.'s fail to tell patients to replenish their bodies with lactobacillus acidophilus and bifidus, (the friendly bacteria).

Lactobacillus Bifidus
The intestines of an infant are free from putrefactive bacteria.

At the beginning of his research, Professor Tessier of Paris, studied bad bacterial invasion of the intestines of young infants. He found that intestines of recently born infants are swarming with putrefactive bacteria. Within a few days, however, the putrefactive bacteria disappeared. Of course, these were breast-fed babies. He states:

Taking their place were particularly shaped acid-forming microbes: Lactobacillus Bifidus. As long as Lactobacillus Bifidus continues to multiply in the intestines of the child, the child enjoys good health. Significantly, the stools of that infant have no offensive odor, only a slight sourness.

As the child begins to eat table food - meat, pasteurized, homogenized milk, processed foods, and sugars - the child's stool begins to have a putrid odor. The putrefactive bacterium multiplies, and the lactobacillus bifidus, which came from the mother's milk, diminishes.

Then the child's sickly journey begins: colds, runny noses, ear infections, fever, and so forth.

Foul-smelling fecal matter is an indication of putrefactive bacteria. Decay is taking place right inside our wonderful bodies. Clients with this symptom can be sure they do not have the friendly bacterium lactobacillus bifidus, which can be replenished in the system either orally or through

193

solutions introduced by an implant after internal cleansing. — IT IS THAT SIMPLE.

Putrefactive Bacteria

With the right balance of favorable bacteria and coliform bacteria, cleansing and correct diet, bowel movements should have no odor.

I am sure you have heard you should cut down on meat because it is bad for you.

I tell my clients it is mucus forming and has no fiber. Bad bacteria thrive on mucus. Because animal products have no fiber, it can lodge in the colon and rot.

Putrefactive bacteria absorb into the body. The minute an animal is killed, putrefaction multiplies in the flesh. Even though you may cook this flesh, not all the bad bacteria are destroyed.

The flesh eaten, putrefactive bacteria get absorbed into the bloodstream. The bacteria eventually destroy the liver, kidneys, and other body-cleaning organs. This process finally leads to serious disease.

Candidiasis

Candidiasis is a relatively newly recognized bowel ailment. Its symptoms are varied and often confused with other maladies. Too often, misinformed doctors dismiss the symptoms as psychosomatic - all in the head of the sufferer.

Candidiasis comes from the Latin word "candida." It is an opportunistic yeast that proliferates in the body when "good" bacteria are absent. It produces toxins along with the overpopulating "bad" bacteria, with consequent ill effects on the body.

Testimonial

Allergy Relief

In this successful case, the claim was made that life-long, serious allergies were relieved through

194

internal cleansing and a detoxification-cleansing program.

This is Mark's R.'s story:

Almost all of my life I have suffered from allergies and asthma, slobbering my way through college and my career.

As if that was not enough, by the time I turned eighteen, I had developed symptoms of candidiasis, including constant fatigue, constipation, bloating, and the feeling that I was never quite digesting my food. Other symptoms included a new case of food allergies and exaggerated allergies to the environment, plus a numbing case of "brain fog," where I was unable to concentrate on any given task of the moment.

For the next twelve years, I went from doctor to doctor, seeking relief from all of these symptoms. In return for such professional medical consultations, I received everything from treadmill tests and blood tests to the latest topical nasal and asthma sprays. Of course, when the doctors discovered that the tests showed nothing and the drugs were not effective, the next role for the doctors to play was psychiatrist. They fired at me questions like, "Are you happy with your job?" and "How often do you have sex?"

With that kind of medical attention, my future looked bleak. Fortunately, I was able to find one allergist who got me started on allergy shots and a rotational diet. The diet was excellent because it eliminated flour and dairy products. I was finally getting some allergy relief.

Several months after starting the allergy shots, my nasal passages had still not cleared enough for easy breathing (You run a great health risk being a mouth breather all of your life. You never know what insect you may inhale!). So, the same doctor kept pushing me to have surgery to correct a mildly deviated septum and my inflamed nasal membranes. I was convinced of the benefit and decided to go ahead with the surgery. The results? A big fat NOTHING!

I consulted acupuncturists and chiropractors. I opted to go ahead with internal cleansing because it seemed to be the most hopeful of my options in getting rid of candidiasis.

After my second session, feeling very light on my feet, I went for a jog in the neighborhood, running the course that I always do. I was delighted to discover that I did not have to stop midstream to catch my breath. I had energy to spare! What's more, I ran home with no asthma attack, which was something new. Sometime after my third session, I was beginning to learn from personal experience the relationship between a clean, functioning colon and clear nasal passages. It seems that clear breathing is proportional to the proper movement of the colon. What an incredible discovery! I wonder how many other allergy problems that people have are related to this concept.

Too bad I wasted so much money on nasal surgery that did not help in the least. I am bothered every time I think of the doctor who was so sure that his surgery would work. He is missing a good part of the complete picture of good health. By the end of the fourth session, I noticed a mood swing. My body was screaming "HAPPY," whether or not I wanted to be. After the fifth session, I no longer had asthmatic reactions to foods, and my "brain fog" was lifting.

I am following Millan's recommended "cleansing" program. and with each visit I have some new health achievement to report. Not only are the symptoms of candidiasis disappearing, the allergies and asthma problems are leaving as well. Spring is typically the worst allergy season, but this spring has been the best I have ever had in my life. I believe my "slobbering" allergy days are becoming a thing of the past!

Thank you, Millan, for your patience, wisdom, and personalized care. The only regret I have is that I did not start my recovery program with internal cleansing in the first place.

Signed, Mark R.

Internal cleansing Restores Body's Natural Balance

According to the study I mentioned earlier, internal cleansing promotes the colonization and growth of the proper ratio of intestinal flora. This restores the correct PH of the colon, the relationship between the acid and alkaline. This in turn, helps to eliminate excess gas, keeps the number of toxic bacteria down, and the toxin reducing bacteria, up. It promotes efficient, beneficial digestion and bowel function.

Internal cleansing counteracts the negative effects of antibiotics and environmental pollutants. Since internal cleansing is much more thorough, bathing the whole large intestine up to the point where it meets the small intestine at the ileocecal valve, actually addresses the problems of initial constipation and any other accompanying problems, especially autointoxication.

A Home Implant

Taking lactobacillus acidophilus and bifidus bacteria (which can be purchased from the refrigerated section at a health food store) rectally and vaginally requires that a client do the following routine:

1. Lie down on a bed; fold a thick towel under the buttocks.
2. Lubricate a syringe of a small enema bulb with Vaseline.
3. Fill with tepid distilled water and one-half teaspoon acidophilus, bifidus. I have my female clients squeeze half the contents of the bulb into their vagina first, and then empty the other half into their rectum. My male clients just empty the whole contents into the rectum.
4. Lie down for two to four hours; read a book or magazine, or sleep.

Do this for five consecutive days.

197

This is a wonderful, stressless, unhurried way for the body to absorb the friendly bacterial flora it needs. A person will be refreshed and ready to continue a good night's sleep. This will expedite the way to optimal health and youthfulness. Clients have stated that it gets rid of candida when they have done it.

Testimonial

Health & Peaceful Sleep Restored

Before internal cleansing, I had trouble sleeping. I could not think clearly or talk to people. I lost my train of thought. I had discomfort and pain in my abdomen. I did a series of treatments along with the cleansing program. Now I sleep well, think more quickly, and talk with ease. My pain is gone and I can digest foods much better than before.
Louisa

Coffee Implants
Coffee implants are very beneficial for many reasons. I am happy to offer coffee implants to my fasting clients. The coffee I use is the same as is used at the Gerson Cancer Clinic. I will implant the coffee after colon therapy for 15 minutes, in order for the coffee to completely absorb within the system.

The following is a list of benefits of organic coffee implants.

1. detox liver
2. duplicates red blood cells
3. distribution of oxygen
4. cancer treatment
5. eliminates constipation
6. weight loss
7. improves nutrient absorption
8. reduces bloating

An Enema User's Account

I used to be very ill. I had arthritis and migraine headaches. I was in and out of hospitals. I thought vitamins were only taken to stay well. Before I knew about internal cleansing, I used to do four enemas a day. I was disgusted and discouraged.

I came home one day and decided to throw every unhealthy food out of my cupboards. I never drank coke or Pepsi anymore. When I changed my diet and did the complete cleansing program, the arthritis and the migraine headaches disappeared.

Angelina

CHAPTER FOURTEEN

FASTING

Most people desire to stay young and healthy. Kings would give all their mighty kingdoms for eternal youth, and millionaires would give their last penny. Ponce De Leon traveled across the world to find the fountain of youth.

Yet, before the flood recorded in the Bible, people lived to be as old as 969 years old.

Why do we not have that today? Why do we have so much pain and suffering?

I think it is within everyone's grasp to stay young and healthy. These states of well-being are available for all, no matter how rich or poor.

Testimonial

Old Waste Removed

I spent 3 weeks at a health institute and then I spent 3 weeks at Millan's supervised fasting retreat. I was amazed at all the old waste that eliminated out of my body, while under Millan's supervision. There was absolutely no old matter that eliminated out of my body the whole 3 weeks at the institute. This made me very angry to realize all the money and time wasted and not getting the results I saw under your care. Thank you so much Millan for the care, cleansings and wisdom you displayed during this stay. I will recommend you to everyone I can.

Sincerely, Matthew B.

Physical Fasting

Before I went on my first fast, I used to think people who fasted would easily die of starvation or, at the least, direly damage their bodies.

Such stories are told by those who simply do not know the facts.

Yes, some of my clients experience the healing crisis but that really is a good sign. As previously mentioned, this means the body is releasing toxins and poisons from the body. This process is to be expected.

I tell clients to hang in there, for it is only temporary. In truth, it will lessen in a day or two, and soon "perfect health" becomes the new goal.

In my years as a Colon Hydrotherapist, I have heard many individuals tell me they have fasted and did not do any type of colon cleansing while they did their fast of four days or more. They felt incredible illness and were miserable! I have heard this so many times. Then, the same individuals did another fast for the same duration of time, but this time cleansing their colon with professional colon hydrotherapy. The difference on how they felt was quite amazing. They had hardly any healing crises or discomfort of any kind. I conclude it is very important to cleanse the colon while doing any fasting for any duration of time. The impurities leave the body more effectively, and with the greatest of ease. I'm all for the ease.

Individuals with specific health conditions or ailments should seek out doctors knowledgeable in the area of fasting. I often hear from people, "I am hypoglycemic and, therefore, cannot fast." Or, "I get headaches and dizziness." Everyone does.

When I did my first cleanse back in 1971, doing juice fasting and herbs, only then did my

202

tummy slim down. I am not saying this will happen to everyone, but it did happen to me. This event was truly one of the turning points in my life.

We never see the insides of our bodies, yet our internal self is key to the condition of our health. It communicates our well-being (or lack of it) in external ways - bags under our eyes, the swelling, the obesity, the quick aging, our disposition in how we treat others around us, our mood swings, our irritation at any little thing that others may say to us, our rudeness, our selfishness, our pride. In my opinion, these symptoms could indicate a toxic body.

Authorities on fasting have different opinions on what kind of fast we should do. One may say to fast on water, only, but another may say juices and water only. I am an advocate of the latter, although I have done both. I feel our conditions and environment are too toxic to deal with water fasting only.

On a water fast, the body will very rapidly release toxins from the body, which could result in a tremendous healing crisis. Headaches, fever, flu symptoms, light-headedness, and so forth could result, to the point that would make one feel extremely sick and miserable. This could be unbearable for some. For this reason I advocate green smoothie fasting. This is the reason why supervised hospital fasts existed centuries ago, where the patient was asked to stay in bed for the whole period of time.

With juice fasting my clients do not feel these symptoms as acutely. The body releases toxins, but much slower. They will still benefit tremendously, though.

Doing the juice fasting, along with taking cleansing herbs and internal cleansing is absolutely the most incredible experience they will ever know. How they feel afterwards is the real evidence.

One client stated, "I could actually see fine lines come off my face each day! It's absolutely amazing"!

Paul Bragg, in his book *Miracle of Fasting*, tells of a twenty-one-day fast he went on. On the nineteenth day of his fast, he said when he went to urinate it felt like red hot water passing through him. He had terrible pain.

He recovered the urine, had it examined, and discovered it to be filled with DDT and other pesticides. Had he stopped his fast on the eighteenth day, he would not have eliminated the DDT. It took the full nineteen days of fasting to rid his body of these poisons.

Testimonial

Overcoming Temperature Intolerance

Another client experienced a regain in body temperature regulation:

> *I was born and raised in California and could not tolerate really hot or very cold weather, but since my body has been cleansed I look forward to going to New York in the winter. I find extreme temperatures do not bother me as in the old days.*
>
> *Randy*

I do not recommend my clients go out and immediately start extensive fasts on their own. They begin a one-day juice fast and about one week later they repeat it. Then they eat only fruits, vegetables, grains, legumes, raw nuts and seeds. After a couple of those fasts, they can begin a supervised seven-day fast.

Going off the fast is very important. I have had clients who have done the seven-day juice fast go off with day eight eating only fruits, day nine adding vegetables, and day ten adding grains, legumes, raw nuts and seeds.

Taking cleansing herbs and internal cleansing is very important and beneficial during this time.

Going off a fast incorrectly can do great damage and even cause death. One case of a man, who successfully went on a thirty-day fast to shrink a tumor, came off the fast and ate a rib-eye steak and potatoes, which his daughter had given him.

She was a nurse and was very worried that her father would starve to death with that length of fast. So when he went off the fast, she was ready to stuff him with this type of food.

Having consumed the meal, he died the next day.

I was diagnosed with borderline diabetes in 1971 and have fasted many times with great success. I also know many people with low blood sugar who have done quite well.

Remember, fasting is not the only way to detoxify the body, but it is definitely the quickest, most effective and very best way to stay young and healthy.

Testimonial

Flu Victim's Story of Recovered Health

When I first called your office, a four-week-old flu was still hanging on. I was experiencing pre-menopausal night sweats, and I was about twenty pounds overweight.

Millan, you answered my questions and suggested I come out later that afternoon and give internal cleansing a try. I could hardly believe it when the very next morning all signs of my flu were gone.

I started on the detoxification program and a series of the internal cleansing sessions, taking one every week. Within a period of three months, I had lost the twenty pounds and cleaned enough

205

toxins from my body so that the night sweats had
ceased. My skin looked clearer and my energy level
increased. My own experience has taught me that
internal cleansing and correct eating are the two
most important factors in regaining youth and
health.

Sandra

Many of my clients will eat only fruits
and vegetables two days before their internal
cleansing appointment. At the same time, they
are taking the cleansing herbs. Then, after
their internal cleansing day, they eat only vegetables, fruits, grains (sprouted grain bread),
legumes, and raw nuts and seeds.

They repeat this process either every three
days or once a week. If they choose to juice fast
then I recommend internal cleansing daily for the
full ten days or two weeks.

Boy, what an exciting time that is! Ask any
one of my clients. The results are incredible.

The reason the body starts to release impurities is because the digestive system is not functioning on a fast. Therefore, the body immediately
starts to get rid of all impurities.

It requires energy for the body to remove the
junk. This energy is normally used to digest food.
But since there is no food to digest, the process of
cleansing begins. This is why I tell my clients "no
exercise, except walking."

The purification process is helped along with
wonderful cleansing herbs. These herbs also remove excess mucus in the small intestines where
most of the digestion takes place. It is this toxic
condition together with the excess mucus in the
body that hinders it from assimilating the nutrients from food.

When my clients fast, there is a possibility
they could struggle with hunger for the first seventy-two hours. But I remind them that the mind

controls their body. Taking the cleansing herbs helps tremendously in controlling their hunger.

Another trick often tried is to take two rounded teaspoons of Bernard Jensen's vegetable broth with a little celery salt. This is poured into a large cup of boiling-hot water. If the client likes spicy food, a few drops of Tabasco sauce may be added. Organic "Better Than Bouillon" is a great product.

This mixture is consumed around 3:00 P.M. and again around 5:30 P.M. This kills the appetite immediately.

In *The Miracle of Fasting*, Paul Bragg tells an interesting story of hiring ten husky college athletes to take a hike with him from Furnace Creek Ranch in Death Valley to Stovepipe Wells, about thirty miles in very hot weather.

The men were allowed to eat all the food they wanted, such as bread, cheese, crackers, lunch meat, hot dogs, and salt tablets.

A station wagon transported and accompanied them with this food. Bragg, who was a great-grandfather at that time, only drank room-temperature distilled water, nothing else.

The hike started around 8 a.m. The college boys gobbled the salt tablets and drank the water. At lunchtime, they ate ham and cheese sandwiches and drank sodas.

They all rested thirty minutes after lunch and continued the rugged hike across the hot burning sands. Pretty soon, three of these stout college boys became violently ill and vomited up their food. They got dizzy, turned pale, and became very weak. They could not continue the hike.

The hike continued with the other seven college athletes. As they continued, they drank large amounts of water and took large amounts of salt tablets. Then, suddenly, five of them got stomach cramps and became deathly ill. They also vomited and none of them could continue the hike. At about 4:00 p.m., the last two athletes collapsed and had to be rushed back for medical care.

As Bragg states, he was the only one left and felt as fresh as a daisy. He had been fasting only on water. He finished the thirty-mile hike, camped out in the desert that night, and the next day hiked back to the ranch where the hike had begun, all by himself and without any food or salt tablets.

Can you imagine, this is a great-grandfather dealing with college athletes?

I know that when I fast and cleanse my body I feel like a young, vibrant woman, with so much energy that I literally go from 6:00 a.m. to 10:00 p.m. and never stop for a break.

Thomas Edison stated, "The doctor of the future will give no medicine but will interest his patients in the care of the human frame, in diet and in the cause and prevention of disease." This is the type of doctor I am interested in visiting!

Testimonial

Lost Weight and More Energy

Dear Millan:

I was inspired to send you this letter regarding hydrocolonic therapy and describe how your nutritional guidance has truly changed my life, physically and otherwise. After only 3 sessions and 3 weeks in which I have not consumed white flour, animals, dairy, white sugar, or processed food, I am fitting into jeans that I have not worn in over one and half years. I have never had so much energy. For the past year on my days off, I would lie in my bed and exercise the remote control. I thought, "This is how forty years olds feel...." My husband and I wanted to make a commitment to our health and colon therapy was one of the things we wanted to investigate for ourselves. This has been an exciting adventure for us. Eric, my husband is diabetic and before we came to you his blood sugar numbers were off the charts accompa-

208

Read Up On Fasting

When a person fasts, it is important to read about cleansing and fasting. Some good books are: *Become Younger*, by Dr. Norman Walker; *The Miracle of Fasting*, by Paul Bragg; and Fasting *Can Save Your Life*, by Herbert Shelton.

Extract Drink Restores Woman on Water Fast

There was a woman who went on a water fast and was becoming very weak. Against her will, she was quickly losing a lot of weight. She then started drinking an extract made of celery, beets, carrots, and potatoes.

When she began drinking it, her energy level increased. She felt much better and was able to go back to her employment while she was still fasting.

This case is another reason why I strongly feel water fasting is not the way to go. Our world is too toxic for that.

My clients who choose to take this extract drink can make it themselves. They just chop up the above ingredients and put them into a large jar filled with distilled water. The proportion is one-third vegetables to two-thirds water. The mixture is refrigerated overnight.

The next day, they can drink it (first stirring the vegetables), then leave it in the jar and drink it throughout the day. They make enough for four to seven glasses' worth. This is sufficient for one day's use.

209

Testimonial

Stop Smoking - Fast!

Many of my clients who were smokers tried everything to stop smoking, and then considered a cleansing fast. Clients have said when they fast, their bodies were repulsed from smoking another cigarette. The same occurs with caffeine or drugs. The desire for these substances can leave because the chemicals which cause the cravings have left, releasing the body from these habit forming materials.

The results prove that fasting cleansed my clients' bodies and immediately does the job to get rid of the toxins, poisons, and sewage inside.

That is the reason that I feel very strongly about resting, especially the first three days of a fast. Exercise is a strong no-no. My clients take short walks, to get the circulation and lymph moving towards elimination.

I am an advocate of fasting. I have seen time and again the benefits of fasting.

When one fasts for any length of time, and I am not talking about a one-day fast, I am talking about seven days or more; taking the cleansing herbs and colon cleansing during the fast is absolutely vital. Earlier advocates of fasting also recommended cleansing herbs with internal cleansing.

Did you know that when one goes without food for a period of time the stomach contracts to half its size? For this reason, a person will feel full if too much is eaten after a fast.

When I supervise a fast, I warn clients to be very careful not to overeat after properly going off their fast. They need to be very aware of this precaution. Even though they are eating God-made foods, they never should overdo it.

I tell them to listen to their body. That may sound strange, but if people are aware of the digestion process taking place in their body, they can avoid over-indulgence.

For starters, the stomach is only the size of a fist. Look at the food on the plate. How much is there? If it is more than their fist's worth, the stomach is weakened by the forced enlargement.

It is impossible to fast when a person is around others who do not understand the benefits of fasting. For any long-term fast of seven days or more, professional supervision is absolutely vital. Do not break the fast when feeling sick. Indeed, this is when the body is eliminating toxins. Rather than taking in food at this time, my clients are advised to drink lemon juice and raw honey mixed in a cup of hot water. This beverage hastens the elimination process.

Everybody is in one of the following states of health: no health, poor health, good health, or excellent health. In which condition of health are you?

Testimonial

Cravings for Cigarettes gone

Dear Millan:
Thank you for the internal cleanses I received. At first, I was apprehensive, because I smoke cigarettes and thought it would be hard to stop, however since my cleansings I have had no urge to smoke and have not missed the cigarettes or wanted to smoke. Also, I forgot my Prozac, but I feel no need for that as well. Some of my water retention went down. Millan, you are a walking testimony for your program, looking years younger than you are with lots of energy.

Signed,
Prema D.

Biblically Spiritual Facts

Senior Citizen Christians that are ill may claim spiritual healing and quote all the scriptures related to healing.

Yes, in His mercy, God does heal - there is no getting around that. I have seen God heal many times. I believe in the healing power of Jesus; however, I cannot and will not accept the fact God will heal us continuously when, in fact, we disobey His dietary laws.

In the Old Testament, God has given instructions regarding diet, but we ignore that. Repeatedly, I have talked with seniors and heard all their complaints. I may make a nutritional suggestion, and they totally ignore it.

Did God not give His wisdom in our diet? It is a known fact Seventh-Day Adventists are the longest-living Christians because they heed their diet, for which I commend them. In contrast, it is unfortunate to see other Christians, and my Jewish friends violate God's laws in their diet.

Those laws are applicable for today. For example, it is a scientific fact that pork, shellfish, high fat, high-sugar, and over-processed foods harm our bodies; nevertheless, we disregard this and ask God's blessing on our food, expecting Him to respect our rebellious choices and disregard His dietary laws.

A senior friend of mine has been sick for two years and is claiming a healing, but she will not be healed if she continues to eat garbage food.

She needs to clean up her eating habits. She claims to be under grace, but she is taking scripture out of context. We have to consider all of God's word, the whole of it. But we can make the Bible say just about anything we want it to, right?

On the other hand, I know a wonderful retired pastor named Orville Johnson. He is a senior citizen now, is working daily down at the beaches or downtown area. He deals with the homeless, feeds the poor, ministers to these people spiritually, goes door knocking, and just shares the love of God. He counsels those in need.

This man of God takes daily walks and my daughter says he drives like a teenager. This man is in his nineties.

His diet consists of vegetables, fruits, grains, raw nuts, seeds and legumes. He makes a nut milk (not cow's milk) to put on his cereal. His mind is sharp and alert. Staying clear of pharmaceutical drugs, he prefers to take daily vitamin and mineral supplements. He has a clean colon and is vibrant and healthy.

Incidentally, Daniel 1:12-20 is an excellent illustration of the need to eat healthy foods. Daniel was under siege by the king of Babylon. This king ordered Daniel and others to eat the delicacies and drink the wine, which the king himself ate.

Daniel and his friends refused, consuming only vegetables and water. They convinced the steward in charge to examine him and his friends

213

in ten days and then compare them to those who ate the king's delicacies.

Daniel and his friends physically looked better than the others; moreover, verse 17 states, *"God gave them knowledge and skill in all literature and wisdom, and Daniel had understanding in all visions and dreams."* Next, when the king called all the men in to examine their mental and physical states, he found Daniel and his three friends ten times more fit than all the magicians and astrologers in his realm.

Is this a motivator, or what?

Daniel got more than that. He got revelation about the coming messiah in detail. WOW! I do not think Daniel was expecting all that. God has given us so much, yet we have used so little.

Spiritual Fasting

Fasting and prayer are two wings of the same bird. It is a state of denial to the flesh. The flesh submits, the spirit prevails. Could it be possible that God does not answer certain prayers because we do not fast? That fasting gives control over the wrongs and weaknesses in life that displease God? One who has never fasted has not drawn as close to God as one could.

I believe there is no closer communion, intimacy, and harmony with God, as when one is fasting.

We are definitely more toxic today than in Bible times; for that reason, I especially advocate starting with juice fasting or green smoothies.

Do not worry about observing a total fast (abstinence from all food and water); trust me, God honors a juice fast.

In Mark 2:20, Jesus says His followers will fast when He is taken away from Earth.

Millions of people attend houses of worship, but few are really being used of God. Why is this? It's because we are not fasting enough. I truly believe this!

214

In Joel 2:12-15, God tells us to turn to Him with fasting, weeping, and mourning - to consecrate a fast. His future wrath may even be turned into a blessing.

Now, can you imagine yourself in obedience to God observing a fast, and, afterward, eating garbage food harmful to the body? God forbid! This would be a quick way to kill yourself! One of the greatest writers and definitely one of the most powerful Christians ever was the Apostle Paul. How many times in his life do you think he fasted? He says in 2 Corinthians 11:22 he fasted often.

I believe that for him to write most of the New Testament as he did, Paul had to have fasted many times, just as King David did in the book of Psalms.

When one fasts for any length of time, God's Word becomes much more alive and understood.

This is powerful stuff!! Let us tap into this. I challenge you!

God says, *"And I will sow her for myself in the land. I will have mercy on her who had not obtained mercy, and I will say to those who were not my people, 'YOU ARE MY PEOPLE!' And they shall say, YOU ARE MY GOD!'" (Hosea 2:23).*

Daniel, mentioned in the bible, was another man of God who fasted when making requests of his Creator. He also fasted in repentance for the sins of Israel.

Do you think we could fast for our country? YES!

In so many sermons, pastors say, "Let's pray for a revival." Yet no revival happens. I have heard this preached many times over the years. I agree whole-heartedly this country needs a powerful revival. Why is God not allowing revival?

I have heard pastors state many reasons; however, I believe it is because Christians are not fasting in their prayer lives.

Why is this not happening folks?

I feel it is because Christians want to have the one fleshly pleasure that the church condones: gluttony. Does this vice not satisfy the flesh? Gluttony is wrong, spiritually and physically.

Attend a potluck sometime, and see all kinds of garbage food with no nutritional value but simply prepared for the pleasure of the palate.

1 Corinthians 6:19 says, *"Or do you not know that your body is the temple of the Holy Spirit who is in you, whom you have from God, and you are not your own? For you were bought at a price; therefore, glorify God in your body and in your spirit which are God's."*

Isaiah 58-59 discusses the importance of the attitude of fasting, but it seems that when the Israelites fasted they were not fasting for the right reasons. They were fasting with deceit in their hearts and disobedience to God in their actions.

Evidently, the Israelites fasted, but for all the wrong reasons. They were still doing all the things, which were an abomination to God. They lied, did not seek out the truth, and spoke with empty words. They conceived evil and brought forth iniquity. They were also seeking out their own pleasure and were speaking their own thoughts.

I have seen the same happen today with a lot of people who come to me and are fasting. They abstain from food for all the wrong reasons, yet say they are achieving a higher level of spiritual awareness by this discipline.

I have to disagree and question what spirit they are talking about!

It says in Isaiah we need to be obedient to God, and that obedience is to feed the hungry, clothe the naked, and help the poor who are cast out. Isaiah goes on to say that then God will hear us but instead, people have chosen their own ways or ways of other gods. The God of the Bible says we must love God with all of our heart and to love our neighbor as we love ourselves.

216

The fast that God has chosen will loosen the bonds of wickedness, undo heavy burdens, and let the oppressed go free. This is the attitude we should have in our fasting.

One Person's Fasting Sets an Oppressed Boy Free

In the book, *Only Love Can Make a Miracle*, Mahesh Chavda shares the powerful effect his obedience to God in the area of fasting had on the life of a severely retarded teenage boy named Stevie. Because of overwhelming self-destructive urges, Stevie had beaten his own face to the point of disfigurement. At the institution where Stevie lived, numerous measures had been taken to change his behavior but to no avail. Stevie was tormented constantly by the other children and he was clearly living a miserable existence.

Moved by compassion for this boy, Mahesh prayed to God for help and direction. God gave Mahesh a word of knowledge that Stevie was being influenced by an evil spirit. The Lord told Mahesh the only help for Stevie was for Mahesh to fast and pray.

After fasting for two weeks, Mahesh took Stevie into a private office, told him that Jesus came to release everyone who was in bondage and that God loved him. Mahesh then called in Jesus' name for the "spirit of mutilation" to come out.

The release for Stevie was instantaneous. He visibly changed and relaxed, no longer full of tension. His self-destructive behavior never returned. As Mahesh says:

My experience with Stevie taught me a great deal. It showed me how powerful evil spirits can be in bringing illness and heartache to human beings. It showed me how much more powerful the name of Jesus to free us from their wicked purposes is. It showed me the importance of fasting.

217

Reasons for Spiritual Fasting

Why are we fasting? Are we fasting in obedience to God? Are we under some bondage or oppression? Maybe we need to fast to release or break those yokes that bind, such as gluttony or eating the wrong foods. These self-destructive habits are not pleasing to God.

Instead of seeking out our own pleasure and our own reasons for fasting, perhaps we need to fast for spiritual reasons. We cannot go wrong, because God has ordained fasting.

Another thing to remember is not to broadcast a fast and run around telling everyone.

There is no better way to draw closer to God and intimate, communal relationship than in fasting. When people fast with the right attitude, their flesh and its weaknesses diminish, and their closeness with God is magnified many times.

Talk about power in prayer!

People fast for their own spiritual awareness, a very self-centered reason for fasting. It has nothing to do with reaching out to others or doing the will of God in loving your neighbor as you love yourself, really sacrificing yourself for other people.

Such individuals do not stand up against wrongs in society. They just turn the other way and ignore their responsibility to fight for what is righteous and moral. They do not speak out against the horrors going on in our culture: child and sexual abuse, violence, sexual promiscuity, rape, etc.

Just like in Isaiah's time, there are people who fast yet are disobedient to God's laws.

In Acts, the early Christians fasted for spiritual leading and the direction God would have them go. If you are considering a job change, a ministry, a marriage, or other significant crossroad, God will give you direction when you fast. Let's really examine this #1 all time best-seller, the *Holy Bible*.

In other words, what we are seeking is God's wisdom, not man's. When we fast and pray, He will give us direction.

In Jonah, we read where a whole city fasted and prayed, and the animals fasted as well. The king instructed everyone not to eat or drink. He also proclaimed that everyone should turn from their evil ways and the violence in their hands (That must have been a pretty bad city!).

Would it not be wonderful if all of us got together to pray and fast even for one day for the United States of America.

Moses fasted forty days and forty nights without food or water.

I am not saying to fast for forty days with no water, but could it be possible that if we fasted for only one day, God would honor that? Remember, he is a merciful God!

Fasting denies the flesh and brings us closer to God. It is one of the most marvelous experiences one can obtain. Sadly, I believe there are many of my Jewish friends and Christian brethren who are not participating in this spiritual discipline; then they wonder why there is no victory in their own lives.

Fasting Is Not a Weight-loss Diet

I give this word of warning to clients who have never fasted: please stay away from the scale while fasting. It can be a big enemy, especially while women fast. This can lead to a tendency of "weighing in" every day.

If one does this, as I did the first time I went on a fast, initial weight loss may be noticeable, but it is followed by slight weight gain. This is not uncommon, and, of course, it is not fat being putting on but the body is retaining fluids.

Remember, the female is the one who reproduces; this is God's way of making sure our generations continue, so He protects the woman from famine by retaining these fluids.

219

Despite this, getting on the scale can be very discouraging. Do not forget, however, fasting breaks the vicious cycle of craving fattening foods, eating them, gaining weight, and feeling out of control.

Yes, during fasting, fat is ultimately lost.

Also, it is important to keep in mind that muscle weighs more than fat. So, if one begins an exercise program, the scale will give the impression of weight gain, when, in actuality, one is losing ugly fat.

My advice is to let one's clothing be the guide. I know we women have to be careful to allow nothing to come along and discourage us! Finally, I warn my clients to be very careful not to overeat when they go off their fast. You can get ravenous after a fast.

Testimonial

Victory over Food Cravings

Even men experience a change in their appetite for certain foods. One client, Andrew, writes:

Dear Millan:

Even after only five internal cleansing sessions in an eight-day period, I felt tremendously relieved. My skin cleared up dramatically, bad breath, body odor, and gas have ceased, and constant cravings for various foods have lessened.

I am looking forward to getting five more treatments when I come back from Japan. I feel certain that internal cleansing can benefit any individual with the desire to improve his or her state of health. It does work.

Signed
Andrew

This client's physical appearance started to improve through a program of cleansing and fasting.

Avoiding Temptation
Some experts on fasting say the appetite (for healthy food) will return only after the body has been detoxified and cleansed. That has not been my case. It is true the appetite subsides after seventy-two hours; however, I can get hungry any time during my fasting. Everyone is different.

I advise my clients against watching TV, or going any place where there is food. It is recommended clients stay away from social gatherings where food is served, and even that homemakers retire into their rooms after preparing the meal for their family.

What Happens During a Fast?
Reading the literature or a book on fasting during this time is very important. During a fast, the body is rebuilding cells and tissues as well as regenerating them. The enzymes and nutrients in juices feed the cells and tissues, giving them nourishment. This, in turn, provides energy, well-being, and good appearance.

Testimonial

Migraine Sufferer

Dear Millan:

I have suffered migraine headaches for quite some time. I had gone to a chiropractor for help, but to no avail.

I have gotten four internal cleansing sessions from you and did your cleansing program. I could not get any more because I am now in Chicago with my family. I am writing to tell you my headaches are gone completely. I cannot believe it! It is so wonderful to have a normal life again.

Sincerely, Dan

Dr. Teofilo De La Torre, in his book, *The Process of Physical Purification*, states the following:

*We can compare the body to a huge
sponge, which is saturated with filthy water.
If we want to cleanse and purify a sponge, we
succeed in doing so by:*

1. *Squeezing the sponge so that the dirty
   filthy water is pressed out. This corre-
   sponds to the process of fasting.*
2. *During the fast, the human sponge is
   being squeezed, thus forcing out of the
   body calcareous deposits, toxins, uric
   acid and other waste products.*

*Then, after the sponge has been
squeezed and part of its filth forced out,
if we submerge it in clean pure water,
the sponge will absorb some of this water and become saturated with a cleaner
and purer fluid. But it may have taken
several processes of squeezing the dirty
water out of the sponge and letting it
absorb clean water before we can succeed in removing all the filth from the
sponge. Equally so, it requires several
processes of fasting, followed by re-
absorption, of pure food, water and air,
before the human sponge can be completely purified, health restored and
immunity to disease acquired. Physiological chemists have analyzed the bodies of animal and human beings who
have died from starvation. Their discoveries throw a new light on the physiological process of fasting. According to
Sterling's "Principles of Human Physiology," proportions: Fat 97%, Spleen
63%, Brain and Cord 0%. By these fig-
ures we see that when the body is deprived of food, it does not consume the
tissues of the body in equal proportions
to maintain the body heat and physiological function. Nor do the more active
tissues wear out faster, as it might be
expected. The opposite is true; the most*

active tissues are the ones that lose the least weight during the fast. The intelligence of the body, when deprived of food, oxidizes the least useful tissues first and keeps intact the most vital tissues. Thus, we see fatty tissues being consumed first and in larger proportion (its loss amounting to 97%) while nerve tissue, being the most vitally important, is left intact. This shows that the nerves and brain are the least dependent on food to maintain their normal functions, as indicted by the fact that nerves and brain are left intact up to the time of death from starvation, as well as by the fact that fasting persons preserve their clearness of mind to the time of death.

De La Torre goes on to state: Professor Huxley of England took a family of earthworms and proceeded to feed them as they usually eat. However, in order to make the experiment, he made this exception: he took a member of the family of worms, separated it from the group and fed it in the same manner but with this exception. Professor Huxley submitted this particular worm to short periods of fasting, followed by periods of feeding on the same kind of food given to its brother worms. The results obtained were remarkable, amazing, and almost miraculous. Much more so if we take into consideration the seemingly unimportant difference to which the one worm was submitted, that is, periodic fasting; otherwise, all the worms were living under the same identical conditions. Professor Huxley was very much surprised to see that the single worm submitted to the fast began to shrink in size and grow very small as the fast proceeded. But as soon as feeding was re-

sumed, the worm began to grow very rapidly, NOT AS AN OLD WORM BUT AS A YOUNG WORM. But the amazing fact was that by means of periodic fasts, Professor Huxley succeeded in maintaining the life of the worm 19 times longer than that of its brothers.

Consider the importance of this discovery. Nineteen generations springing up from brother worms had come into being, procreated, declined, and died, while this particular worm (through periodic fasting) had been rejuvenated and was very much alive when Huxley stopped the experiment.

Another observation by Huxley was that worms, animals, or even humans, if fed all the food they wanted and had no work to do, became lazy, fat, infirm, rigid, and grew old before their times.

It has been my observation that when a person fasts periodically, life is extended and one becomes a healthy, energetic, and vivacious individual. This experiment is certainly worth thinking about and considering.

Another study was done on rats of the same litter. One rat was fed all it wanted anytime. His sibling was fasted periodically during its lifetime. The amazing discovery was that the rat that was fasted periodically outlived his sibling 10 times longer!

CHAPTER FIFTEEN

Quote: Anger is a condition in which the tongue works faster than the mind.
Millan Chessman

SENIORS

Seniors

We were not meant to suffer from preventable diseases. Evidence shows that wise health habits can keep us physically fit, mentally alert, and healthy—well into old age.

Some people claim they would not want to live that long. However, dynamic health and vigor might change their minds!

Great health and longevity are not miracles waiting to be discovered by some scientist in the distant future. This is for us today.

How unfortunate to hear a child say, "I don't want to sit next to Grandma—she smells."

Grandmas should be snuggled up to and cuddled with; that is one of the reasons God gave them to us.

One sign of putrefactive bacteria is a foul odor when defecating. The smell is offensive, requiring copious amounts of air freshener to mask the stench. One unfortunate senior lady told me she had to leave her mobile home every time her husband had a bowel movement.

Testimonial

Improved Vision

Read the following account of Bob, a client who experienced renewed eyesight:

My eyes started failing when I was thirteen years old. My prescription glasses got progressively stronger throughout high school, college, and the Navy. I am fifty-one years old now.

Always being nearsighted, I went to vision clinics for years, doing vision exercises and such. But I could not really stop my eyesight from degenerating. I was always trying to get it to improve, but it only worsened. I did a seven-day cleansing program two months ago and did not notice any change. Then I completed another seven-day cleansing program, a five-day cleansing program, and then another seven-day cleansing program. After each cleanse, I tested my eyes on a home eye chart. With this last eye chart testing (wearing my glasses), everything was very blurry, and I could not figure out what was going on. I just changed my prescription recently, and now it seems my glasses are too strong! It is just like magic! This is incredible!

Anonymous

Centenarians

Ripley's Believe It or Not states:

In 1993, a Mrs. Harriet Breedlove of Knoxville, Tennessee was cutting a new set of teeth at the age of 102. Mr. Thomas Gordon of Grand Rapids, Michigan, had his hair turn black at the age of 103. Daphne Travis of Atlanta, Georgia at the age of 108 years was hale and hearty and was cutting the third set of teeth. Her eyesight was improving and her hair, which was white as new wool for 50 years, was turning black again. George Washington Emerson of Newport, Maine, was cutting his third set of teeth at age 93 years.

*He says he is not yet ready to retire; instead,
he wants to go into the chicken business. He
has never been sick except once with measles.
He has never had to wear glasses.*

Many of these centenarians worked until
they died. A few daily walked a good distance,
Ripley explained.

An interesting case was a Chinese man
who lived to be 254 years old. Documentation
verified his age. His lifelong diet was mostly
vegetables, especially herbs and roots. His
name was Lin Ching Wan.

Another centenarian lived to 160. His
birth certificate proved it. Interestingly, this
man fathered his thirty-sixth child at age nine-
ty-six. In later years, he grew black hair and
cut new teeth.

An investigation of these folks reveals their
diet consisted mainly of vegetables, fruit, seeds,
nuts, and grains. Most were vegetarians, eating
these God-made foods.

Before the great flood, recorded in the Bible,
people were vegetarians. After the flood, they had
to eat meat. Now, the average life span is seventy
four years instead of eight hundred.
Individually, we have little control over our environment. We breathe impure air consisting of
carbon dioxide and monoxide. Our insides are
poisoned. Our air loses precious oxygen from
heaters. The list goes on and on.

Testimonial

Healthy Octogenarian
*One 87-year-old client sees me every ten days for
her internal cleansing. After being treated by a
clinic in Tijuana ten years ago for breast cancer,
her cancer went into remission. She became a strict
vegetarian and underwent colon cleansing. She
does internal cleansing regularly for prevention.
Her mind is alert, and she remembers much of her*

past. This dear lady has a lot of energy! Occasionally, she forgets her appointment with me, but, all in all, she is remarkable
Her Name is:
Alice

Downward Spiral to Illness

Yes, our diet may yield a life span of 60, 70 or perhaps 80 years. But it will also produce painful, debilitating, and expensive ailments that now begin around age forty-five, and will plague the hapless body until death.

We all share the picture of senile, wheelchair-bound, or bedridden old age, with the sufferer consigned and forgotten in some inadequate nursing home and awaiting a meaningless, painful, and humiliating death. These decrepit people are simply weakened by disease, decay, and a degeneration of cells and tissues of the body.

A number of years ago, I used to take little children to visit old folks in convalescent homes as a ministry.

So many were abandoned by their families. Many were unkind and crabby. Some were so decrepit they looked frightening! You know what they gave them for snacks? Cookies and milk—such a constipating combination. Sadly, the residents cannot say, "no, thank you." They have but one choice: to eat what is given them. Perhaps this is "physical endurance," but it is certainly not living with a high quality of life. A piece of fresh fruit, or a glass of freshly squeezed juice rather than the milk and cookies, would be a healthier choice.

I saw one old woman who, in her desperation to defecate, was trying to take out stool with her fingers! Is this what we can expect in our last days? God forbid!

Chillingly, statistics are pointing to an earlier onset of the "diseases of old age" in our society, and our expected life span may be shrinking. Bad health originating in an unhealthy colon poisoned by bad diet is the culprit.

228

Too many of us have resigned ourselves to the idea that age brings disease, sloth-like behavior, and disorientation. Take a look back through these pages at the testimonies of people whose lives were dramatically changed through internal cleansing and proper diet, and then at the studies cited which implicate that a bad diet is a leading cause in virtually all types of diseases.

Folks, good health really starts with a better diet and internal cleansing. A good mental attitude and an exercise program are valuable partners in a comprehensive health program, but they do not equal the importance of eating the right foods. Eating the right foods is the number one priority for attaining and maintaining optimal health.

Dr. Norman Walker, one of the grandfathers of modern internal cleansing, wrote seven books on health and colonics. A personal friend, who knew him quite well, once told me that when Walker died in 1987, he was 118 years old. To this day, he is respected and honored by those in preventive health. Walker advocated colon cleansing - sometimes daily for six weeks. Generally, the usual recommendations are around ten sessions, including an herbal cleansing program with a modification of diet.

Look at the convalescent hospitals. What a shame that their residents are not contributing their experiences and wisdom to young people. This is a tragedy for our society.

If we would eat God-made foods (plant-base diet), instead of man-made foods, and stop taking drugs for every ache and pain (with all of drugs' side effects), society would not have to stick its elderly away in old folks' homes, out of sight, out of mind. Go to a convalescent home and look around. Smell the decay everywhere.

I want to be an asset to my grandchildren and great-grandchildren, with all the wisdom and experience God has given me. I want to be an asset to others way into my eighties and nineties eventually, perhaps even dying in my sleep.

In my old age and in obedience to God, I want be a blessing to others.

Far too many older people in churches and synagogues are not healthy. I recently had lunch with a senior, whom I have known for a number of years. She is very ill with every ache and pain imaginable and is quite obese. She treats her body like a garbage can. She eats whatever she thinks tastes delicious and does not consider what is nutritious. More than that, she does not stop to consider God's plan for her health.

This individual has been sick for two years and she is expecting God to heal her. I do not think she realizes it makes a fool out of God to think He is always going to heal when we violate our bodies.

Seniors' Dilemma

Many elderly folks are so caught up in their own physical pain and suffering, they cannot be involved in charity or show concern for others. How can they when they themselves are hurting so much?

Usually, they are taking many prescription drugs, which compound their problems which traps them into a vicious cycle. They want to do God's will, but they simply cannot - they are too sick.

Remember the last time you were sick? You were so involved in yourself, right? You could care less about anything else. These senior citizens are in this state of mind.

CHAPTER SIXTEEN

Quote: When we control the body, we give freedom to His Spirit. Millan Chessman

COLONICS AND ENEMAS

A Better Way: Colon Hydrotherapy

A better way is a complete internal cleansing program.

It is gentle, painless, and odorless. It is clean and dry. It is relaxing and you have the opportunity to learn nutritional information from your colon hydrotherapist during the procedure. It is comfortable - you can lie down and take a break. It is not humiliating—you will not fail. It is not embarrassing; my clients are totally covered. It is not undignified. There is no discomfort. It is not stressful. My clients even receive an abdominal massage! Afterwards, my clients feel vibrant and are on their way to better health.

In contrast to the minimal standards required for enemas, colon hydrotherapy's standards are high. We use state-of-the-art, name-brand equipment mounted next to the table, where the client lies during the procedure. This internal cleansing equipment is capable of controlling water pressure, temperature, and flow.

The equipment features a clear glass, florescent-lighted view tube. Through this, any discharge is observed and examined. The tube is also a direct disposal line for toxins and stool. All speculum and hoses are disposable.

231

Properly trained Colon Hydrotherapists

Clients must be very careful that their colon hydrotherapists are fully qualified, certified, and recommended by others. I cannot emphasize enough, the importance of a properly trained, certified colon hydrotherapist.

One client told me she had gone to a so-called colon hydrotherapist to have therapy. First, the therapist inserted the speculum. She then turned the client over on her back, and began to turn the water on. The client then asked her what she was doing: "Are you aware that this speculum is in my vagina?" The therapist described above was no bargain! Clients should seek colon hydrotherapists who demonstrate the utmost concern for the health and well-being of clients rather than bargaining-table proposals. A properly educated, certified colon hydrotherapist is imperative.

If you are interested in learning the profession of Colon Hydrotherapy, you may contact my daughter's school, California Coastal Cleansing Institute phone 760-918-0030. She has been a Colon Therapist since 1986 and is the best.

Character Requirements

Colon hydrotherapy is administered by a certified, trained colon hydrotherapist. The procedure requires no drugs. First, a small speculum is gently inserted by the client into their body. To encourage peristalsis, water is slowly introduced until the need for evacuation is felt. The colon then eliminates the water along with the waste.

Empathy for the patient is required. A sensitive therapist enables patients to relax. Kindness, gentleness, being soft-spoken, and caring for people are vital qualities in a colon hydrotherapist.

A colon hydrotherapist must discern the needs of the client. Therefore, the colon hydrotherapist must be a knowledgeable and skilled specialist.

Soothing Water

Today, colon hydrotherapists know that filtered and sanitized water at body temperature is best for administration of internal cleansing. It does not irritate the colon; therefore, it is not harmful. The client hardly feels the water going in, and with a knowledgeable, professional colon hydrotherapist, the cleansing is a comfortable procedure.

Testimonial

Colonics Made a Difference in Her Health

Dear Millan:

I appreciated very much the help and concern that you lovingly extended to me. It made such a big difference at such a critical time of my life. You are truly a godly woman, and I have much respect for you. The 21 colonics I received from you did indeed help my health. I learned so much. The colonics made a difference. Thank you again, Millan.I have more energy and my skin cleared up.

Signed,
Debbie S.

Proper Equipment

We need to understand how important it is that water enters the body very slowly. Water entering the colon too fast would stimulate peristalsis too soon and cause discomfort.

The only known cases of perforation of the colon occurred in hospitals (which involved infants, and mentally disturbed patients) with adults administering enemas, not colon hydrotherapy. These are the reasons professional internal cleansing equipment is superior to that of an enema. With proper equipment, the water temperature can be controlled and kept at a comfortable 90 to 105 degrees Fahrenheit.

Relaxing and Gentle

There is no discomfort, no offensive odors, and no mess. The client does nothing; the equipment does all the work.

At my office, clients provide their health history and discuss with me their health needs, concerns, and the general state of their current health. I have treated children as young as six years old, and those as old as ninety-four years.

The colon hydrotherapist puts the client at ease by attending to questions, explaining functions of the equipment, and, using charts on the wall, describing how the procedure is done. Reassuring the client of her (most colon hydrotherapists are women) gentleness is important.

Testimonial

Pneumonia Gone

Dear Millan:

My ten-year-old son was diagnosed with bronchial pneumonia. The doctors insisted he be hospitalized immediately.

Since I have not benefited from the medical system in the past, I refused and decided to have him receive ten sessions from you along with your cleansing program. After the fourth treatment, all symptoms of his pneumonia were gone.

He is eating healthy foods now and feels great. Thank you for being so gentle and loving towards my son.

Anonymous

The Actual Therapy

When a client arrives at the colon hydrotherapist's office, he or she is escorted into the bathroom and given a hospital gown. The client removes all clothes from the waist down, except socks.

234

The client at this time empties the bladder completely.

It is imperative that the colon hydrotherapist is working with modern, name-brand equipment, outfitted with safety features, and sanitation with ultraviolet light. It may also contain various implants prescribed by a physician, such as an implant container and oxygen therapy.

Many health practitioners believe that more oxygen can be absorbed through the colon than through the lungs. This oxygen gets absorbed into the bloodstream and bathes the cells in the body.

She must monitor the progress of the colonic cleansing, massage the client's colon through the abdomen, and satisfactorily explain the procedure of cleansing the colon. Lymphatic massage during the therapy can be administered as well. The colon therapist should explain what she is doing and what is happening in the digestive tract.

Just before administering the colon hydrotherapy, the ileocecal valve must be correctly closed by the therapist. This is to prevent any fecal matter or toxins in the colon from "engrossing" or being back flushed (allowed back into the small intestine).

Once the ileocecal valve is securely closed, the client lies on the right side, drawing knees to chest in the fetal position. By this time, the client feels comfortable with the therapist.

It is very important that the colon hydrotherapist not only be knowledgeable but also be gentle and caring. The client will assist in inserting the speculum.

The insertion should be completely painless.

When the speculum is in place, the colon hydrotherapist helps the client roll over onto the back. Again, knees are bent, but feet are flat on the table.

The client's hospital gown ensures complete coverage.

When the client is comfortable and everything is in place, the process begins.

The disposable speculum is only ½ inch in diameter and rests comfortably in the rectal area. The speculum not only delivers water into the colon, it also removes the water and the waste, as two separate hoses are attached to the other end of the speculum.

The colon hydrotherapist turns on the water gradually. The water temperature is the same as the body temperature. Most people do not even notice the water because of this, and so agree that this is a smooth and comfortable procedure. The colon hydrotherapist will pulsate the output tube as she administers the internal cleansing. The client may not even feel this, since it is comfortable. The purpose of the pulsation is to loosen fecal matter in the lower end of the bowel by simulating peristaltic waves. Pulsating the output tube also helps by preventing too much water from getting behind and around the feces.

If the client has excess gas, it takes a little longer for the stool to eliminate. The water cannot get past the gas and travel further up the colon.

At each session, both client and colon hydrotherapist will observe dislodged waste floating through the view tube, which is contained in the equipment.

Often during a session, I cannot help exclaiming to clients, "Look at what you are eliminating!"

The two of us then closely examine the contents flowing through the well-lighted tube. We may notice blotchy brown clouds, flecks, and more solid matter of black, brown, or even yellow. Sometimes the discharge is ropy-looking or has ridges. I have even seen hair and tablets tumbling down the view tube during a session.

Sometimes it is necessary for the client to sit on the toilet to expel (this is very rare, as the equipment is most often capable of doing the job).

Muscle tone of the colon is judged by the vigor of expulsion and the vibration of the observation tube as noted by the therapist. There could be slight cramping, similar to that of menstrual cramps (which also can be helped through internal cleansing). The cramping simply means the colon is going back in the shape it should be in. That is why we call this "colon hydrotherapy"; we are actually doing therapy on the colon muscle.

During a single colon cleansing session the client's colon hydrotherapist typically fills and evacuates the water four or more times. Many people benefit from at least ten cleansing sessions of about forty-five minutes each. They have commented on experiencing a state of health, vigor, youthfulness, and well-being.

An attractive young woman was correcting her eating habits, but still had bowel movements only once every seven days or so. During her first session, the water could not reach past the sigmoid, just above the rectum; her colon was that badly impacted.

That happens sometimes because of a lifetime of poor eating habits. A good diet alone cannot easily tone a flaccid, toxic colon.

I instructed her to sit on the toilet and eliminate. It took an extended series of cleansings, during which all the impacted sewage was expelled. The results of the cleansing indicated that, she was doing just fine.

After a session of thirty minutes to an hour, the water passing through the view tube usually becomes bubble free and clear.

Newcomers to the procedure are often apprehensive, as we all are of the unknown. But before long, they feel comfortable with the protocol and think nothing of it.

They are smiling and relaxed.

There is no pain, no personal anxiety, only soothing conversation and gentle massage, interesting viewing, and perceptible health benefits.

When the procedure is finished, the speculum is gently and slowly withdrawn by the client.

Totally covered, the client is rolled again onto the back and helped to a sitting position. At this time, it is common to feel a little stiff from lying in the same position for an hour. Clients take this opportunity to limber up a little.

Next, the colon hydrotherapist helps the client down from the table to go into the bathroom, eliminate, and get back into street clothes. By this time, most people feel reinvigorated, light-footed, and full of bouncy energy. Remember you are getting a bath inside of your body for the first time in your life.

Chronic illness can be a thing of the past. When your body is clean, your immune system is raised and is better able to combat viral attacks from outside the body, rather than fighting toxins produced by the garbage rotting inside .

Testimonial

Ultra Marathon Runner Came in Second

I followed your cleansing program and colon cleansing for two weeks. I am an ultra-marathon runner, and after completing the fasting and colon cleansing, I bulked up for another two weeks to prepare for the Western States one-hundred-mile race.

At that time, I put back on the weight I had lost during the two-week cleanse. Out of all of the runners, I came in second in that race. Of all the races I have run, I have never come that close to coming in first. I had incredible energy after my cleanse. Thank you.

Anonymous

Internal cleansing: An Inexpensive, Simple Procedure

An hour of internal cleansing at the current rate is quite reasonable, considering all one gets for the money. It is a simple, relaxing procedure

238

where the recipient lies comfortably and has a safe washing of the colon.

There is no expensive operating room or multiple trained staff; no needles, band-aids, scrubs, shaves, scalpels, or anesthesia; no cutting, sawing, breaking, clamping, stitching, or stapling; no time in a recovery room, no cold room temperature to bring your temperature and blood pressure down, and no prosthetics.

The result is surprisingly pleasant. Even after the first treatment, the client feels much better.

There are no drugs or prescriptions to fill afterward that could possibly become addictive and certainly have side effects. No blood lost, transfused, or soiling skin and clothes. No yellow or purple stains from antiseptic washes and markings. No bruising, deep tissue damage or nausea.

I have asked many doctors what causes cramping during internal cleansing, and they all give different answers. I believe it is because the colon most likely has some narrow areas. It is the movement of the cleansing herbs and stool, expanding the colon walls through these passages, that causes discomfort. A gastroenterologist I know agreed.

A head pressure of one foot could cause water to reach the cecum in two to five minutes with professional equipment. This will not happen with someone that has a spastic colon or colitis. When the cecum is chronically irritated, some health practitioners suspect the client to have conditions such as the following: arthritis, sinusitis, tonsillitis, or infection.

A toxic colon can overwork the liver, causing the liver to enlarge, and lead to a congested liver. This condition would be indicated by a colon displacement at the hepatic flexure as shown on an X-ray.

It is very important that a client not eat food two hours before the colonic cleansing appointment so there is no digestion going on during the

239

colonic. The client may drink small amounts of liquids such as juice, herb teas, and water. The client may eat afterwards.

I have had clients tell me that after their treatment they were ravenous, not for junk food but for a salad or other healthy meals.

It is so wonderful to know that internal cleansing can stop the vicious cycle of craving garbage food or compulsive overeating.

I have heard of many therapists who insert hot water (body temperature, of course) and then reduce the temperature, stating the cold water will cause peristalsis in the colon.

I do not believe this is good for the client and have found it really does not achieve promised results. Dr. Harvey Kellogg, in his book *Colon Hygiene,* states this practice can be very painful and should be discouraged.

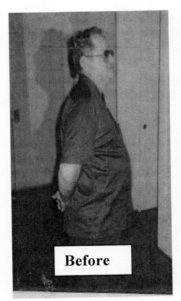
Before
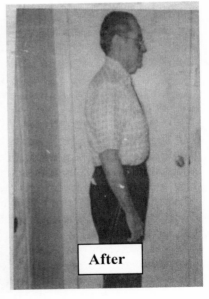
After

This client's physical appearance improved through my program of internal cleansing.

Free From Medications!

For 5 years, I have been in and out of doctor's offices, complaining about sharp pains by my right side. The doctors put me on different prescribed medications. Nothing helped. They all told me it was irritable bowel syndrome, for which they said there is no cure. They said it was due to stress. I spent literally three to five thousand dollars in about four years on medications - all to no avail! Recently, my chiropractor suggested internal cleansing. Even after the first session, I felt 80% better. I'm now on my 7th session, and have continued relief. My bowels now move more regularly without any of the pain I've experienced before. I highly recommend internal cleansing to everybody.

Signed, Lisa

Enemas

In my home cleansing program, the booklet includes easy instructions on how to do an enema comfortably, correctly and effectively to achieve the best results.

Some hospitals still give enemas. Even a minimally skilled aide can administer one. Time-consuming, potentially messy, and requiring certain cleanup preparations, the procedure is avoided whenever possible.

In general, professional colon hydrotherapy differs totally from and lacks the offensive stigma of enemas.

Thus, the economic tide turned from costly personnel's administration of colon cleansing. The result was from 1960 to the present, the majority of the medical doctors stopped prescribing colon hydrotherapy and reduced the use of enemas. There was never any proof established that enemas were harmful or worthless, it just was not cost-effective.

Enema Solutions
In the early 1900's, gastroenterologists sometimes recommended enema solutions of soapsuds, salt, molasses, soda, vinegar, sugar, oil of turpentine, and other harmful materials. It seems they did not understand these substances would irritate the mucus membranes of the colon. One medical doctor, H. Kellogg, in his book *Colon Hygiene*, recommended sour milk enemas in cases of colitis, chronic constipation, diarrhea, excessive gas, chronic appendicitis, and chronic diarrhea. In Kellogg's testing of five hundred people, he discovered that only fifteen percent had good bacteria in their colons. Why such a low count? Because we destroy good bacteria by eating too much sugar, caffeine, alcohol, animal products, and taking medications such as antibiotics!

A Natural Enema
When my clients cannot get to a colon hydrotherapist, and are feeling discomfort, I suggest the following recipe produces excellent results:

1/2 pint of molasses
1/2 pint warm, distilled water

Mix solution and use in an enema bag to flush out the colon.

This natural enema is harmless and very agreeable with the colon. Another way my clients evacuate their colons is to lie on their backs and gently knead their lower abdomens with their fists.

Testimonial

Asthma Gone and 33 pounds lighter

Dear Millan:
In the past there were several times when my asthma was so severe that I needed to take emergency action to save my life. I am now truly a believer in the importance of internal cleansing for detoxifying the body, and nutrition for building up

242

the immune system after seeing the results and changes in my health since cleansing. Now four months later, I am 33 pounds lighter and everyone compliments me on how I appear to glow with good health. I have remained off my oral medication, no longer use steroid inhalers, and now I only use albuterol inhaler as needed. I have become such a walking testimony to the benefits of internal cleansing that my sister and brother-in-law, as well as my mother and father have gone through the series of internal cleansing as well. What a difference internal cleansing has made in my life. I am truly grateful to the Lord for prayers answered regarding my health, and that He led me to you.

Adrianne W.

CHAPTER SEVENTEEN

Quote: The power of the tongue controls the words we say and the condition of our health. Millan Chessman

WATER

Drinking Distilled Water vs. Mineral Water

In his book, *The Truth about Water*, Paul Bragg describes his personal experience with numerous watermelon flushes. He says on several occasions he ate nothing but watermelon and drank watermelon juice for ten days.

Typically, during that period, he would take a sample of the first urine voided in the morning. He then would seal the container tightly and shelve it for six months to one year.

Because he is a biochemist, he would thoroughly analyze this substance. He found calcium and magnesium carbonate and other inorganic minerals had been expelled in this urine.

If these inorganic minerals were beneficial to the body's health, they would not be voided during any kind of cleansing. The only thing our bodies expel when cleansing are deleterious poisons.

Toxic acid crystals and inorganic minerals can cause hardening of the arteries, which leads to strokes, arthritis, heart attacks, etc.

Bragg shares a story about a man who went to a hot mineral water resort to take mineral baths. There, it was suggested he drink the mineral water because it was good for him and his body needed the minerals.

Bragg discouraged the man from drinking the water, but his advice was ignored. For six months, the man drank this mineral water.

One night, during his stay at the resort, people heard him scream in agonizing pain. When they reached him, he was dead.

An autopsy showed a large kidney stone puncturing a large artery is what killed him.

The primary chemical in Splenda, as well as artificial sweeteners, is now showing up in municipal water supplies. Like too many other things the FDA approves, it was never tested properly, Chlorine doesn't break it down and it passes right through the system into our water supply.

I personally believe in drinking distilled water only, not spring or mineral water. There are many arguments about which is better. After investigating all the pros and cons and from my own experience, I conclude in favor of distilled water.

Besides, it tastes much better than any other water. Also, it can be purchased at any grocery store. Or, better yet, one may invest in a distiller and produce home-distilled water.

People may write me, and I will be happy to direct them to where they may buy one for a reasonable price.

Those in favor of mineral water state that it has valuable minerals, which are necessary for the body. But, it must be remembered, these are inorganic minerals, the same as found in dirt. If people were starving and began to eat the dirt with these inorganic minerals, they would soon die.

These minerals do not assimilate into the body for utilization. They actually do damage, in that they are deposited into the joints, gall bladder, and other parts of the body. Organic minerals are very necessary for our bodies to function well, not inorganic minerals.

Incrustation in pipes is caused by inorganic mineral water. Similarly, kidney stones are a result of drinking mineral water.

If they investigate the authorities' opinions on which water to drink (I am talking about those who have researched this subject themselves),

245

they will unanimously conclude that drinking distilled water is vital to good health. For further information, read Paul Bragg's book, as mentioned above.

Testimonial

An RN's Health Improved

Dear Millan:
> *I wanted to express my appreciation to you for helping me move in the direction of better health. Working as an RN at San Diego Hospice, I've had the experience of seeing many individuals suffer. Many times I've thought if only they had access to a health practitioner like you. What if colon hydrotherapy were part of their treatment plan. Would their prognosis have been different? After receiving a series of ten treatments from you and following the detox program, my overall health, energy level, and well-being has improved. My overall skin is clear for the first time in years. Thank you so much, Millan.*

Sincerely,
Cindy T. RN

I need to tell you my story. When I was in my thirties, I would travel up and down the coast, once a month, to visit my family, who lived in Monterey. Half way through the trip, I would have to stop and stretch my legs because I would get this pain behind my hip bone. I don't know what it was but it was relieved when I stretched my legs. This happened every time I took long trips and sat for a long period of time. I did that for about five years, then I would travel to Monterey four times a year.

About three and a half years ago, at 68 years old, I started getting the same pain quite regularly, traveling back and forth to Julian. It became worse and worse, that every time I sat for twenty minutes or more and stood up – the pain

246

was so excruciating that I would feel like I could not walk and then it would subside gradually. It became noticeable with my family because I would end up limping and I actually thought I was going to be a cripple and would need a cane. My husband and children became very concerned. In desperation, I decided to see a medical doctor. They did x-rays and could not find anything wrong. I then went to a chiropractor and their treatments did not do any good and last of all I went to a naturopathic physician. He gave me a shot in that area, hoping it would resolve the pain problem – it did not. This went on for approximately one year.

I then heard about F. Batmanghelidj, M.D. and watched his DVD on water. At the time, I was drinking one liter a day, thinking that would be all I needed. Dr. Batmanghelidj stated we need to drink at least two liters of water a day. He also stated in his research that people who have pain in their bodies, would find that the pain would disseminate after drinking this required amount of water. Of course, my ear perked up and I thought, "I got to give this a try."

I started drinking two liters of water each day, and on the third day, the pain was gone and never returned. At this writing, I am totally pain free.

Drinking water at the correct time maximizes its effectiveness on the Human body:

a) 2 glasses of water after waking up helps activate internal organs

b) 1 glass of water 30 minutes before a meal - helps digestion

c) 1 glass of water before taking a bath - helps lower blood pressure

d) 1 glass of water before going to bed - avoids stroke or heart attack.

Benefits of drinking two liters of water are:
1) it will reduce your appetite
2) it will assist in bowel elimination
3) it will keep the kidneys clean
4) it will increase energy at times of lethargy
5) it intensifies detoxification of the body
6) it reduces pain.

NOTES

Millan's Tips for Excellent Health

1. Eat mostly fruits and vegetables, as much raw as possible. Lightly steamed vegetables are okay.

2. Cut out foods with additives, preservatives, as well as processed, refined and enriched.

3. Remove all refined white sugar from your diet. Replace it with raw honey, stevia, raw sugar, rice syrup, real maple syrup, barley malt and xylitol also.

4. Eliminate all animals from your diet, including eggs.

5. Remove all white flour foods from your diet. Replace with sprouted grain, stone ground, whole wheat or seven grain. Read labels – if it says "enriched" don't eat it. Try Ezekiel 4:9 breads.

6. Only eat fats from the following food items: Avocado, raw nuts, seeds, olives, and flax seed oil, and virgin olive oil. All of these will flush out fat from your fat cells and have other benefits as well. Roasted nuts and seeds make you fat.

7. Do not eat pasteurized, homogenized dairy. Instead, eat raw cheese, soy yogurt, or soy ice cream. *Silk Brand* products are very tasty. Eat only organic soy products.

8. Exercise! Break a sweat each day with an aerobic activity. Start gradually by walking at a comfortable pace, at least four times a week. Then continue to add minutes and

variety to your walks or other forms of exercise.

9. Get a good night's sleep. If you have insomnia, be sure to cut out caffeine, alcohol, and take liquid minerals. See Millan for available products or visit, www.coloniccleanse.com.

10. Drink one quart of green smoothies daily, consisting of organic spinach, spring mix, kale, celery, cucumbers and other greens, mixed with 1/2 frozen banana and 3 dates, all blended together. This will give you more energy and a better night sleep, I promise. I do this every single day!!

11. Fast 24 hours once a week. Drink only juices and water. The easiest way to fast is by having a large meal around noon, and then don't eat again until the next day at noon.

12. Cleanse semi-annually or annually. This includes taking cleansing herbs, colonics, and modification of the diet.

13. Drink eight, 8 oz. glasses of distilled water daily to curb appetite and give you energy.

Begin to Restore Your Health Now!
The bad news in health is a nasty, clogged-up colon.

The good news is it can be cleaned and good health restored.

And it is not such a scary thing to do!

Almost everybody who comes to me comes back for more internal cleansing as a regular preventive, like taking their car in for required maintenance checkups. Without them, the car's performance fails.

Without a clean colon, one's health fails..

Many people, who were initially nervous, embarrassed and even frightened to death at the prospect of the complete internal cleansing program got over it and come back again and again. Because of how they look and feel, they know what they are doing is for their own good.

I always try to convey to my clients my empathy, care, concern, gentleness, and love. They know I am here to help them live long, happy, healthy, and productive lives.

So how about you?

What are you waiting for?

Since more and more people are turning to the services of Colon Hydrotherapy, I would like to emphasize the need for more professional Colon Hydrotherapists. There is such a demand in this field. This profession is growing by leaps and bounds.

If you are interested in learning the profession from the best in the field, my daughter Roxanne Watson has a school here in San Diego and is a qualified Instructor through International Association for Colon Therapy.

FOR INQUIRIES AS TO OUR PRODUCTS, CLEANSING PROGRAM, AND MILLAN'S FASTING RETREAT CONTACT:

MILLAN CHESSMAN
2633 Windmill View
El Cajon, CA 92020
619-562-5446
Website: www.coloniccleanse.com
Email: millanchessman@gmail.com

BIBLIOGRAPHY

American Colon Therapy Association, *Research Project.*

Anderson, Richard, *Cleanse & Purify Thyself,*

Ariola, Paavo, *Rejuvenation Secrets from Around the World,*

Bragg, Paul, *Miracle of Fasting*
Truth About Water.

Christopher, John, M.D., *Three Day Cleansing Program and Mucusless Diet,*

Chavda, Mahesh, *Only Love Can Make a Miracle,*

De la Torre, Teofilo, M.D., *Process of Physical Purification,*

Ehret, Professor Arnold, *Mucusless Diet Healing System; Rational Fasting.*

F. Batmanghelidj, *MD Health Miracles in Water and Salt*

Gray, Robert, *Colon Health Handbook.*

Great Smokies Laboratory.

Kellogg, John Harvey, M.D. *Colon Hygiene*

Knox, D.C., J. Glenn,

Lewkovich, D.C., Gary.

Louis, David, *2201 Fascinating Facts*

Malmstromm, Dr. Crister Inged.

252

Mantell, M.D., Donald J., "Hydrotherapy and Its Clinical Applications,"
Pare, Dr., Writings from 1600 A.D.

Ripley's Believe It or Not!

Shelton, Herbert M., *Fasting Can Save Your Life.*

Tesslor, Dr. Gordon, *Lazy Person's Guide to Better Nutrition.*

Vegetarian Times,

Waddington, M.D., Joseph, *Scientific Intestinal Irrigation and Adjuvant Therapy.*

Walker, Norman, D.C., *Become Younger.*

Wells, William, *The Shocking Truth About Cholesterol.*

Wilkerson, Jim, KGTV Channel 10 News

Wiltsie, M.D., James W. *Antique Colonic Machine taken from Chronic Intestinal Toxemia and its Treatment.*

CPSIA information can be obtained at www.ICGtesting.com
Printed in the USA
LVOW101141260212

270476LV00001B/2/P